Dash Diet Cookbook 2019 for Beginners:
500 Quick, Easy and Healthy Dash Diet Recipes
21 Day Dash Diet Meal Plan to Lose Weight and Lower Your Blood Pressure

Tina Cooper

ISBN: 9781693611636

Table of Content

Introduction

Before diving into the recipes themselves, let's talk a little bit about the program itself!

About the DASH Diet

"DASH" is an acronym for (Dietary Approach To Stop Hypertension), which is essentially a diet program that was designed to help individuals with hypertension or high blood pressure to help control their condition.

However, you should understand that aside from helping control your blood pressure, the DASH diet program comes with a plethora of other health benefits too!

Unlike many other diets out there that ask you to get rid of almost all of your favorite food groups, the DASH diet tends to follow a different pathway and asks you to control the "daily serving" of certain foods as opposed to eliminating them from your regime.

Perhaps one of the more exciting aspects of the Dash Diet is the fact that this particular diet is perhaps one of the very few that have been approved and promoted by the U.S Department of Health and Human Services. So, you can rest easy, knowing that this is not just another fad diet!

The DASH Diet helps to deal with your hypertension directly by inspiring you to lower your sodium intake and eat food that is healthier and richer in potassium.

And just in case you don't know, potassium helps to lower the effects of sodium, which again, helps to lower down blood pressure, and that allows your body to experience a plethora of health benefits.

While the DASH diet primarily focuses on increasing the intake of fruits, vegetables, and low-fat dairy items, you are still allowed to go for meat-based recipes, although in small quantities.

Keeping that in mind, the recipes found in this book are a combination of all sorts of recipes, ranging from simple vegetarian to exquisite meat recipes, to ensure that you have a plethora of options to choose from!

How to enter the program

Entering the DASH program is pretty easy, and the general outline is as follows:
- 6-8 servings of whole grains (daily)
- 4-5 servings of vegetable (daily)
- 4-5 servings of fruits (daily)
- 2-3 servings of low-fat dairy (Daily)
- 6 or fewer servings of lean meat, poultry or fish (daily)
- 2-3 servings of healthy fats/oils (daily)
- 4-5 servings of nuts, seeds, and legumes (weekly)
- 5 or fewer servings of sweets (weekly)

While we have already provided a sample meal plan with this book, you might be tempted to come up with the meal plan that suits you. So, if you intend doing that, make sure you follow the outline above.

You should understand that a single serving of rice will not be the same as a single serving of potatoes, even though both of them are from the same group.

If all goes well, you should get results just after 2 weeks, and just in case you are wondering how you should make the changes to your regular diet to enter Dash Diet, well:

Keep in mind that the number of servings depends on how many calories you need per day, which will change depending on your sex, weight, etc.

An excellent way to calculate your daily calories is to use free online calorie calculators.

Once you have decided your calorie intake, start your DASH diet by making incremental and gradual changes.

- An excellent way to start is to limit your sodium to 2,400 mg per day and reduce it eventually
- Once your body has adjusted itself to the change, go for 1,500 mg per day (which is about 2/3 spoon)

(Keep in mind that the sodium count includes both the sodium already present in your food as well as any additional salt that you might add.)

So, to summarize -

- Consume more fruits, low-fat dairy foods, and vegetables
- Try to cut back on foods that are high in cholesterol, saturated fat and trans fat
- Eat whole-grain foods, nuts, poultry and fish
- Try to limit sodium, sugary drinks, sweets and red meat, such as beef/pork, etc.

And you should be good to go!

How does the DASH diet promote weight loss and exercise?

Despite not being specifically designed for weight loss, the Dash Diet does indeed help to trim down your weight through various indirect means.

While the DASH diet does not stress reductions in calories, it does influence you to fill up your diet with very nutrient-dense food as opposed to calorie-rich food, and this easily helps to shed a few pounds!

Since you will be on a heavy diet of veggies and fruits, you will be consuming lots of fiber, which is also believed to help in weight loss.

Aside from that, the diet also helps to control your appetite since cleaner and nutrient-dense foods will keep you satisfied throughout the day! Lower food intake will further contribute to weight loss.

And while you are at it, the program will indirectly encourage you to carry out a daily workout to keep your body healthy and fit. Following the DASH Diet program while working out will significantly enhance the effectiveness of the program.

Understanding the food groups

To keep things simple, let me break down the food groups so that you can understand the food regime of the program better.

Eat as much as you want

- Grains, such as barley, wheat bread, wheat pasta, etc.
- Meats, such as eggs, lean beef, lean chicken, lean pork
- Seafood, such as fish, Shrimp, and Salmon
- Fruits such, as apples, bananas, cherries, grapes, blackberries, mangoes, etc.
- Vegetables such as artichokes, broccoli, Brussels sprouts, carrots, bell peppers, green beans, etc.

Limit Your Servings

- Healthy vegetable oils, such as canola, corn, olive, etc.
- Condiments
- Dairy such, as Greek yogurt, skim milk, low-fat milk, low-fat cheese
- Nuts, legumes, and seeds such as almonds, cashews, flax seeds, hazel nuts, lentils, pecans, kidney beans
- Red meats

Eat Rarely

- Sweets such as beverages, jams, jellies, sugars, sweet yogurt
- Saturated fats such as bacon, cholesterol, coconuts, fatty meats
- Sodium rich foods such as canned fruits, canned vegetables, gravy pizza, etc.

Understanding daily proportions

Controlling your daily portions is crucial when it comes to the Dash Diet program. While the key component here is to keep your sodium intake at a low level, there are other things that you must consider.

So, to properly maintain your DASH diet, you should:

- Consume more fruits, low-fat dairy foods, and vegetables
- Try to cut back on foods that are high in cholesterol, saturated fat and trans fat
- Eat more whole-grain foods, nuts, poultry and fish
- Try to limit sodium, sugary drinks, sweets and red meat, such as beef/pork, etc.

Research has shown that you will get results within just 2 weeks!

Alternatively, a different form of diet known as DASH-Sodium calls for cutting down sodium to about 1,500 mg per day (which weighs about 2/3 teaspoon per day)

Generally speaking, the suggested DASH routine includes:

- Daily 7-8 servings of grains
- Daily 4-5 servings of vegetables
- Daily 4-5 servings of fruits
- Daily 2-3 servings of low-fat/ fat-free dairy products
- Daily 2 or less servings of meat/fish/poultry
- 4-5 servings per week of nuts, dry beans, and seeds
- Daily 2-3 servings of fats and oil
- Less than 5 servings per week of sweets

And just to give you an idea of what "Each" serving means, here are a few pointers.

The following quantities are to be considered as 1 serving:

- ½ cup of cooked rice/pasta
- 1 slice of bread
- 1 cup of raw fruit or veggies
- ½ cup of cooked fruit or veggies
- 8 ounces of milk
- 3 ounces of cooked meat
- 1 teaspoon of olive oil/ or any healthy oil
- 3 ounces of tofu

Some salt alternatives to know about

Letting go of salt might be a little bit difficult for people who are going into this diet for the first time.

To make the process a little bit easier, here are some great salt alternatives that you should know about! Some of them are used in the recipes in our book, and you may use them if needed.

Sunflower Seeds

Sunflower seeds are amazing salt alternatives, and they give a nice nutty and slightly sweet flavor. You may use the seeds raw or roasted.

Fresh Squeezed Lemon

Lemon is believed to be a nice hybrid between citron and bitter orange. These are packed with Vitamin C, which helps to neutralize damaging free radicals from the system.

Onion Powder

For those of you who don't know, onion powder is a dehydrated and ground spice that is made out of onion bulb. The powder is mostly used for seasoning in many spices! Keep in mind that onion powder and onion salt are two different things.

We are using onion powder here. They sport a nice mix of sweet, spice and a bit of an earthy flavor.

Black Pepper Powder

The black pepper powder is also a salt alternative that is native to India. You may use them by grinding whole peppercorns!

Cinnamon

Cinnamon is a very well-known and savory spice that comes from the inner bark of trees. Two varieties of cinnamon include Ceylon and Chinese, and they sport a sharp, warm and sweet flavor.

Flavored Vinegar

Fruit-infused vinegar or flavored vinegar, as we call it in our book, is a mixture of vinegar that is combined with fruits to give a nice flavor. These are excellent ingredients to add a bit of flavor to meals without salt. Experimentation might be required to find the perfect fruit blend for you.

As for the process of making the vinegar:

- Wash your fruits and slice them well
- Place ½ cup of your fruit in a mason jar
- Top them up with white wine vinegar (or balsamic vinegar)
- Allow them to sit for 2 weeks or so
- Strain and use as needed

The awesome health benefits

Now, before you move forward, let me share some of the awesome health benefits that you are going to enjoy while you are on the program.

Lower Blood Pressure

This is perhaps the main reason why the DASH diet was even invented!

Salt is believed to be very closely related to increasing blood pressure. The purpose of the DASH diet is to closely monitor the intake of salt and reduce it to very minute levels and improve your overall blood pressure.

Aside from the salt itself, the DASH diet also helps to control the levels of potassium, magnesium, and calcium, which altogether plays a great role in lowering blood pressure as well!

The balanced diet also helps to control cholesterol and fat levels in your system, which prevents atherosclerosis, which further helps to keep the arteries healthy and strain-free.

Helps Control Diabetes

Since the Dash Diet helps to eliminate empty carbohydrates and starchy food from your diet while avoiding simple sugars, a fine balance between the glucose and insulin level of the body is created that helps to prevent diabetes.

Also:

- Lowers blood pressure
- Helps to lower cholesterol levels
- Helps in weight loss (discussed later)
- Gives you a healthier heart
- Helps to prevent Osteoporosis
- Helps to improve kidney health
- Helps to prevent cancer
- Helps to control Diabetes
- Helps to prevent depression

Sample 21-Day Meal Plan

Now, keep in mind that the following plan is crafted to give you an idea of how you might develop your plan. Since the caloric requirement varies from one person to the next, your plan might be different than the one provided here.

Regardless, make sure to consult with your nutritionist before coming up with your very own plan.

Week 1	Breakfast	Lunch	Dinner
Sunday	Healthy Zucchini Stir Fry	Chicken and Carrot Stew	Hearty Garlic and Kale Platter
Monday	Power-Packed Oatmeal	Epic Mango Chicken	A Green Bean Mixture
Tuesday	Chia Porridge	Spicy Cabbage Dish	Authentic Zucchini Boats
Wednesday	Hearty Pumpkin Oats	Excellent Acorn Mix	Roasted Onions and Green Beans
Thursday	Power-Packed Oatmeal	Epic Mango Chicken	A Green Bean Mixture
Friday	Chia Porridge	Spicy Cabbage Dish	Authentic Zucchini Boats
Saturday	Hearty Pumpkin Oats	Excellent Acorn Mix	Roasted Onions and Green Beans

Week 2	Breakfast	Lunch	Dinner
Sunday	**Coconut Porridge**	**Balsamic Chicken and Vinegar**	**Hearty Ginger Soup**
Monday	**Barley Porridge**	**Humble Mushroom Rice**	**Coconut Arugula Soup**
Tuesday	**Hearty Pineapple Oatmeal**	**Sweet and Sour Cabbage and Apples**	**Minty Avocado Soup**
Wednesday	**Delightful Berry Quinoa Bowl**	**Delicious Aloo Palak**	**Butternut and Garlic Soup**
Thursday	**Coconut Porridge**	**Balsamic Chicken and Vinegar**	**Hearty Ginger Soup**
Friday	**Barley Porridge**	**Humble Mushroom Rice**	**Coconut Arugula Soup**
Saturday	**Hearty Pineapple Oatmeal**	**Sweet and Sour Cabbage and Apples**	**Minty Avocado Soup**

Week 3	Breakfast	Lunch	Dinner
Sunday	**Banana Steel Oats**	**Delicious Garlic Tomatoes**	**Onion Soup**
Monday	**Banana and Buckwheat Porridge**	**Spicy Kale Chips**	**Broccoli and Tilapia**
Tuesday	**Vanilla Sweet Potato Porridge**	**Almond Buttery Cabbage Dish**	**Fennel and Almond Bites**
Wednesday	**Avocado and Blueberry Medley**	**Brussels Fever**	**Cauliflower Bagels**
Thursday	**Banana and Buckwheat Porridge**	**Spicy Kale Chips**	**Broccoli and Tilapia**
Friday	**Vanilla Sweet Potato Porridge**	**Almond Buttery Cabbage Dish**	**Fennel and Almond Bites**
Saturday	**Avocado and Blueberry Medley**	**Brussels Sprouts Fever**	**Cauliflower Bagels**

- If you feel hungry in-between meals, try to go for some snacks if you like. This is fine as long as you don't exceed your caloric requirement.

Chapter 1: Breakfast Recipes

Cinnamon and Coconut Porridge

Serving: 4

Prep Time: 5 minutes

Cook Time: 5 minutes

Ingredients:

- 1 cup water
- 1/2 cup 36-percent low-fat cream
- ½ cup unsweetened dried coconut, shredded
- 1 tablespoon oat bran
- 1 tablespoon flaxseed meal
- 1/2 tablespoon almond butter
- 1 ½ teaspoons stevia
- ½ teaspoon cinnamon
- Toppings, such as blueberries or banana slices

How To:

1. Add the ingredients to a small pot and mix well until fully incorporated
2. Transfer the pot to your stove over medium-low heat and bring the mix to a slow boil.
3. Stir well and remove from the heat.
4. Divide the mixture into equal servings and let them sit for 10 minutes.
5. Top with your desired toppings and enjoy!

Nutrition (Per Serving)

- Calories: 171
- Fat: 16g
- Protein: 2g
- Carbohydrates: 8g

Coconut Porridge

Serving: 2
Prep Time: 15 minutes
Cook Time: Nil
Ingredients:

- 2 tablespoons coconut flour
- 2 tablespoons vanilla protein powder
- 3 tablespoons Golden Flaxseed meal
- 1 ½ cups almond milk, unsweetened
- Powdered Erythritol

How To:

1. Take a bowl and mix in the flaxseed meal, protein powder, coconut flour and mix well.
2. Add the mix to the saucepan (placed over medium heat).
3. Add almond milk and stir, let the mixture thicken.
4. Add your desired amount of sweetener and serve.
5. Enjoy!

Nutrition (Per Serving)

- Calories: 259
- Fat: 13g
- Carbohydrates: 5g
- Protein: 16g

Cinnamon Pear Oatmeal

Serving: 2
Prep Time: 10 minutes
Cook Time: 15 minutes
Ingredients:

- 3 cups water
- 1 cup steel-cut oats
- 1 tablespoon cinnamon powder
- 1 cup pear, cored and peeled, cubed

How To:

1. Take a pot and add the water, oats, cinnamon, pear and toss well.
2. Bring it to simmer over medium heat.
3. Let it cook for 15 minutes, and divide into two bowls.
4. Enjoy!

Nutrition (Per Serving)

- Calories: 171
- Fat: 5g
-
- Carbohydrates: 11g
- Protein: 6g

Banana and Walnut Bowl

Serving: 4
Prep Time: 10 minutes
Cook Time: 15 minutes
Ingredients:

- 2 cups water
- 1 cup steel-cut oats
- 1 cup almond milk
- ¼ cup walnuts, chopped
- 2 tablespoons chia seeds
- 2 bananas, peeled and mashed
- 1 teaspoon vanilla flavoring

How To:

1. Take a pot and add all ingredients, toss well.
2. Bring it to simmer over medium heat.
3. Let it cook for 15 minutes, and divide into 4 bowls.
4. Enjoy!

Nutrition (Per Serving)

- Calories: 162
- Fat: 4g
- Carbohydrates: 11g
- Protein: 4g

Scrambled Pesto Eggs

Serving: 2
Prep Time: 5 minutes
Cook Time: 5 minutes
Ingredients:

- 2 large whole eggs
- 1/2 tablespoon almond butter
- 1/2 tablespoon pesto
- 1 tablespoon creamed coconut almond milk
- Sunflower seeds and pepper as needed

How To:

1. Take a bowl and crack open your eggs.
2. Season with a pinch of sunflower seeds and pepper.
3. Pour eggs into a pan.
4. Add almond butter and introduce heat.
5. Cook on low heat and gently add pesto.
6. Once the eggs are cooked and scrambled, remove from the heat.
7. Spoon in coconut cream and mix well.
8. Turn on the heat and cook on LOW for a while until you have a creamy texture.
9. Serve and enjoy!

Nutrition (Per Serving)

- Calories: 467
- Fat: 41g
- Carbohydrates: 3g
- Protein: 20g

Barley Porridge

Serving: 4
Prep Time: 5 minutes
Cook Time: 25 minutes
Ingredients:

- 1 cup barley
- 1 cup wheat berries
- 2 cups unsweetened almond milk
- 2 cups water
- Toppings, such as hazelnuts, honey, berry, etc.

How To:
1. Take a medium saucepan and place it over medium-high heat.
2. Place barley, almond milk, wheat berries, water and bring to a boil.
3. Lower the heat to low and simmer for 25 minutes.
4. Divide amongst serving bowls and top with your desired toppings.
5. Serve and enjoy!

Nutrition (Per Serving)

- Calories: 295
- Fat: 8g
- Carbohydrates: 56g
- Protein: 6g

Olive Cherry Bites

Serving: 30
Prep Time: 15 minutes
Cook Time: Nil
Ingredients:

- 24 cherry tomatoes, halved
- 24 black olives, pitted
- 24 feta cheese cubes
- 24 toothpick/decorative skewers

How To:
1. Use a toothpick or skewer and thread feta cheese, black olives, cherry tomato halves in that order.
2. Repeat until all the ingredients are used.
3. Arrange in a serving platter.
4. Serve and enjoy!

Nutrition (Per Serving)

- Calories: 57
- Fat: 5g
- Carbohydrates: 2g
- Protein: 2g

Roasted Herb Crackers

Serving: 75 Crackers
Prep Time: 10 minutes
Cook Time: 120 minutes
Ingredients:

- ¼ cup avocado oil
- 10 celery sticks
- 1 sprig fresh rosemary, stem discarded
- 2 sprigs fresh thyme, stems discarded
- 2 tablespoons apple cider vinegar
- 1 teaspoon Himalayan sunflower seeds
- 3 cups ground flaxseeds

How To:

1. Preheat your oven to 225 degrees F.
2. Line a baking sheet with parchment paper and keep it on the side.
3. Add oil, herbs, celery, vinegar, sunflower seeds to a food processor and pulse until you have an even mixture.
4. Add flax and puree.
5. Let it sit for 2-3 minutes.
6. Transfer batter to your prepared baking sheet and spread evenly, cut into cracker shapes.
7. Bake for 60 minutes, flip and bake for 60 minutes more.
8. Enjoy!

Nutrition (Per Serving)

- Calories: 34
- Fat: 5g
- Carbohydrates: 1g
- Protein: 1.3g

Banana Steel Oats

Serving: 3
Prep Time: 10 minutes
Cook Time: 15 minutes
Ingredients:

- 1 small banana
- 1 cup almond milk
- ¼ teaspoon cinnamon, ground
- ½ cup rolled oats
- 1 tablespoon honey

How To:

1. Take a saucepan and add half the banana, whisk in almond milk, ground cinnamon.
2. Season with sunflower seeds.
3. Stir until the banana is mashed well, bring the mixture to a boil and stir in oats.
4. Reduce heat to medium-low and simmer for 5-7 minutes until the oats are tender.
5. Dice the remaining half of banana and put on the top of the oatmeal.
6. Enjoy!

Nutrition (Per Serving)

- Calories: 358
- Fat: 6g
- Carbohydrates: 76g
- Protein: 7g

Swiss Chard Omelet

Serving: 2
Prep Time: 5 minutes
Cook Time: 5 minutes
Ingredients:

- 2 eggs, lightly beaten
- 2 cups Swiss chard, sliced
- 1 tablespoon almond butter
- ½ teaspoon sunflower seeds
- Fresh pepper

How To:

1. Take a non-stick frying pan and place it over medium-low heat.
2. Once the almond butter melts, add Swiss chard and stir-cook for 2 minutes.
3. Pour the eggs into the pan and gently stir them into the Swiss chard.
4. Season with garlic sunflower seeds and pepper.
5. Cook for 2 minutes.
6. Serve and enjoy!

Nutrition (Per Serving)

- Calories: 260
- Fat: 21g
- Carbohydrates: 4g
- Protein: 14g

Hearty Pineapple Oatmeal

Serving: 5
Prep Time: 10 minutes
Cook Time: 4-8 hours
Ingredients:

- 1 cup steel-cut oats
- 4 cups unsweetened almond milk
- 2 medium apples, sliced
- 1 teaspoon coconut oil
- 1 teaspoon cinnamon
- ¼ teaspoon nutmeg
- 2 tablespoons maple syrup, unsweetened
- A drizzle of lemon juice

How To:

1. Add listed ingredients to a cooking pan and mix well.
2. Cook on very low flame for 8 hours/or on high flame for 4 hours.
3. Gently stir.
4. Add your desired toppings.
5. Serve and enjoy!
6. Store in the fridge for later use; make sure to add a splash of almond milk after re-heating for added flavor.

Nutrition (Per Serving)

- Calories: 180
- Fat: 5g
- Carbohydrates: 31g
- Protein: 5g

Zingy Onion and Thyme Crackers

Serving: 75 crackers
Prep Time: 15 minutes
Cooking Time: 120 minutes
Ingredients:

- 1 garlic clove, minced
- 1 cup sweet onion, coarsely chopped
- 2 teaspoons fresh thyme leaves
- ¼ cup avocado oil
- ¼ teaspoon garlic powder
- Freshly ground black pepper
- ¼ cup sunflower seeds
- 1 ½ cups roughly ground flax seeds

How To:

1. Preheat your oven to 225 degrees F.
2. Line two baking sheets with parchment paper and keep it on the side.
3. Add garlic, onion, thyme, oil, sunflower seeds, and pepper to a food processor.
4. Add sunflower and flax seeds, pulse until pureed.
5. Transfer the batter to prepared baking sheets and spread evenly, cut into crackers
6. Bake for 60 minutes.
7. Remove parchment paper and flip crackers, bake for another hour.
8. If crackers are thick, it will take more time.
9. Remove from oven and let them cool.
10. Enjoy!

Nutrition (Per Serving)

- Total Carbs: 0.8g
- Fiber: 0.2g
- Protein: 0.4g
- Fat: 2.7g

Crunchy Flax and Almond Crackers

Serving: 20-24 crackers
Prep Time: 15 minutes
Cooking Time: 60 minutes
Ingredients:

- ½ cup ground flaxseeds
- ½ cup almond flour
- 1 tablespoon coconut flour
- 2 tablespoons shelled hemp seeds
- ¼ teaspoon sunflower seeds
- 1 egg white
- 2 tablespoons unsalted almond butter, melted

How To:

1. Preheat your oven to 300 degrees F.
2. Line a baking sheet with parchment paper, keep it on the side.
3. Add flax, almond, coconut flour, hemp seed, seeds to a bowl and mix.
4. Add egg white and melted almond butter, mix until combined.
5. Transfer dough to a sheet of parchment paper and cover with another sheet of paper.
6. Roll out dough.
7. Cut into crackers and bake for 60 minutes.
8. Let them cool and enjoy!

Nutrition (Per Serving)

- Total Carbs: 1.2
- Fiber: 1g
- Protein: 2g
- Fat: 6g

Basil and Tomato Baked Eggs

Serving: 2
Prep Time: 10 minutes
Cook Time: 15 minutes
Ingredients:

- 1/2 garlic clove, minced
- 1/2 cup canned tomatoes
- ¼ cup fresh basil leaves, roughly chopped
- 1/4 teaspoon chili powder
- 1/2 tablespoon olive oil
- 2 whole eggs
- Pepper to taste

How To:

1. Preheat your oven to 375 degrees F.
2. Take a small baking dish and grease with olive oil.
3. Add garlic, basil, tomatoes chili, olive oil into a dish and stir.
4. Crack eggs into a dish, keeping space between the two.
5. Sprinkle the whole dish with sunflower seeds and pepper.
6. Place in oven and cook for 12 minutes until eggs are set and tomatoes are bubbling.
7. Serve with basil on top.
8. Enjoy!

Nutrition (Per Serving)

- Calories: 235
- Fat: 16g
- Carbohydrates: 7g
- Protein: 14g

Cool Mushroom Munchies

Serving: 2
Prep Time: 5 minute
Cook Time: 10 minutes
Ingredients:

- 4 Portobello mushroom caps
- 3 tablespoons coconut aminos
- 2 tablespoons sesame oil
- 1 tablespoon fresh ginger, minced
- 1 small garlic clove, minced

How To:

1. Set your broiler to low, keeping the rack 6 inches from the heating source.
2. Wash mushrooms under cold water and transfer them to a baking sheet (top side down).
3. Take a bowl and mix in sesame oil, garlic, coconut aminos, ginger and pour the mixture over the mushrooms tops .
4. Cook for 10 minutes.
5. Serve and enjoy!

Nutrition (Per Serving)

- Calories: 196
- Fat: 14g
- Carbohydrates: 14g
- Protein: 7g

Banana and Buckwheat Porridge

Serving: 2
Prep Time: 10 minutes
Cook Time: 15 minutes
Ingredients:

- 1 cup of water
- 1 cup buckwheat groats
- 2 big grapefruits, peeled and sliced
- 1 tablespoon ground cinnamon
- 3-4 cups almond milk
- 2 tablespoons natural almond butter

How To:

1. Take a medium-sized saucepan and add buckwheat and water.
2. Place the pan over medium heat and bring to a boil.
3. Keep cooking until the buckwheat absorbs the water.
4. Reduce heat to low and add almond milk, stir gently.
5. Add the rest of the ingredients (except the grapefruits).
6. Stir and remove from the heat.
7. Transfer into cereal bowls and add grapefruit chunks.
8. Serve and enjoy!

Nutrition (Per Serving)

- Calories: 223
- Fat: 4g
- Carbohydrates: 4g
- Protein: 7g

Delightful Berry Quinoa Bowl

Serving: 4
Prep Time: 5 minutes
Cook Time: 15 minutes
Ingredients:

- 1 cup quinoa
- 2 cups of water
- 1 piece, 2-inch sized cinnamon stick
- 2-3 tablespoons of maple syrup

Flavorful Toppings

- ½ cup blueberries, raspberries or strawberries
- 2 tablespoons raisins
- 1 teaspoon lime
- ¼ teaspoon nutmeg, grated
- 3 tablespoons whipped coconut cream
- 2 tablespoon cashew nuts, chopped

How To:

1. Take a metal strainer and pass your grain through them to strain them well.
2. Rinse the grains under cold water thoroughly.
3. Take a medium-sized saucepan and pour in the water.
4. Add the strained grains and bring the whole mixture to a boil.
5. Add cinnamon sticks and cover the saucepan.
6. Lower the heat and let the mixture simmer for 15 minutes to allow the grain to absorb the liquid.
7. Remove the heat and fluff up the mixture using a fork.

8. Add maple syrup if you want additional flavor.
9. Also, if you are looking to make things a bit more interesting, just add any of the above-mentioned ingredients.

Nutrition (Per Serving)

- Calories: 202
- Fat: 5g
- Carbohydrates: 35g
- Protein: 6g
- Protein: 1.4g

Fantastic Bowl of Steel Oats

Serving: 4
Prep Time: 5 minutes
Cook Time: 25 minutes
Ingredients:

- 3 ¾ cup water
- 1 ¼ cup steel-cut oats
-
- ¼ teaspoon salt

Flavorful Toppings

- 1 teaspoon cinnamon
- ½ teaspoon nutmeg
- ½ teaspoon lemon pepper
- 1 teaspoon Garam masala
- Mixed berries as needed
- Diced mangos as needed
- Sliced bananas as needed
- Dried fruits as needed
- Nuts as needed

Flavorful Toppings

- 1 tablespoon coconut milk

How To:

1. Take a medium-sized saucepan and bring it over high heat.
2. Add water and allow the water to heat up.
3. Add the steel-cut oats with some salt and lower the heat to medium-low.
4. Let the mixture simmer for about 25 minutes, making sure to keep stirring it all the way.
5. Add coconut milk or almond butter for some extra flavor.
6. Once done, serve with some berries or nuts.
7. Enjoy!

Nutrition (Per Serving)

- Calories: 125
- Fat: 3g
-
- Carbohydrates: 20g
- Protein: 7g

Quinoa and Cinnamon Bowl

Serving: 2
Prep Time: 10 minutes
Cook Time: 15 minutes
Ingredients:

- 1 cup uncooked quinoa
- 1½ cups water
- ½ teaspoon ground cinnamon
- ½ teaspoon sunflower seeds
- A drizzle of almond/coconut milk for serving

How To:

1. Rinse quinoa thoroughly underwater.
2. Take a medium-sized saucepan and add quinoa, water, cinnamon, and seeds.
3. Stir and place it over medium-high heat.
4. Bring the mix to a boil.
5. Reduce heat to low and simmer for 10 minutes.
6. Once cooked, remove from the heat and let it cool.
7. Serve with a drizzle of almond or coconut milk.
8. Enjoy!

Nutrition (Per Serving)

- Calories: 255
- Fat: 13g
- Carbohydrates: 33g
- Protein: 5g

Awesome Breakfast Parfait

Serving: 2
Prep Time: 5 minutes
Cook Time: Nil
Ingredients:

- 1 teaspoon sunflower seeds
- ½ cup low-fat milk
- 1 cup all-purpose flour
- 1 teaspoon vanilla
- 3 eggs, beaten
- 1 teaspoon baking soda
- 2 cups non-fat Greek yogurt

How To:

1. Break up pretzels into small-sized portions and slice up the strawberries.
2. Add yogurt to the bottom of the glass and top with pretzel pieces and strawberries.
3. Add more yogurt and keep repeating until you have used up all the ingredients.
4. Enjoy!

Nutrition (Per Serving)

- Calorie: 304
- Fat: 1g
- Carbohydrates: 58g
- Protein: 15g

Amazing and Healthy Granola Bowl

Serving: 6
Prep Time: 5 minutes
Cook Time: 25 minutes
Ingredients:

- 1-ounce Porridge oats
- 2 teaspoons maple syrup
- Cooking spray as needed
- 4 medium bananas
- 4 pots of Caramel Layered Fromage Frais
- 5 ounce fresh fruit salad, such as strawberries, blueberries, and raspberries
- ¼ ounce pumpkin seeds
- ¼ ounce sunflower seeds
- ¼ ounce dry chia seeds
- ¼ ounce desiccated coconut

How To:

1. Preheat your oven to 300 degrees F.
2. Take a baking tray and line with baking paper.
3. Take a large bowl and add oats, maple syrup, and seeds.
4. Spread mix on a baking tray.
5. Spray coconut oil on top and bake for 20 minutes, making sure to keep stirring from time to time.
6. Sprinkle coconut after the first 15 minutes.
7. Remove from oven and let it cool.
8. Take a bowl and layer sliced bananas on top of the Fromage Fraise.
9. Spread the cooled granola mix on top and serve with a topping of berries.
10. Enjoy!

Nutrition (Per Serving)

- Calories: 446
- Fat: 29g
-
- Carbohydrates: 37g
- Protein: 13g

Cinnamon and Pumpkin Porridge Medley

Serving: 2
Prep Time: 10 minutes
Cook Time: 15 minutes
Ingredients:

- 1 cup unsweetened almond/coconut milk
- 1 cup of water
- 1 cup uncooked quinoa
- ½ cup pumpkin puree
-
- 1 teaspoon ground cinnamon
- 2 tablespoons ground flaxseed meal
- Juice of 1 lemon

How To:

1. Take a pot and place it over medium-high heat.
2. Whisk in water, almond milk and bring the mix to a boil.
3. Stir in quinoa, cinnamon, and pumpkin.
4. Reduce heat to low and simmer for 10 minutes until the liquid has evaporated.
5. Remove from the heat and stir in flaxseed meal.
6. Transfer porridge to small bowls.

7. Sprinkle lemon juice and add pumpkin seeds on top.
8. Serve and enjoy!

Nutrition (Per Serving)

- Calories: 245
- Fat: 1g
- Carbohydrates: 59g
- Protein: 4g

Quinoa and Date Bowl

Serving: 2
Prep Time: 10 minutes
Cook Time: 15 minutes
Ingredients:

- 1 date, pitted and chopped finely
- ½ cup red quinoa, dried
- 1 cup unsweetened almond milk
- 1/8 teaspoon vanilla extract
- ¼ cup fresh strawberries, hulled and sliced
- 1/8 teaspoon ground cinnamon

How To:

1. Take a pan and place it over low heat.
2. Add quinoa, almond milk, cinnamon, vanilla, and cook for about 15 minutes, making sure to keep stirring from time to time.
3. Garnish with strawberries and enjoy!

Nutrition (Per Serving)

- Calories: 195
- Fat: 4.4g
- Carbohydrates: 32g
- Protein: 7g

Crispy Tofu

Serving: 8
Prep Time: 5 minutes
Cook Time: 20-30 minutes
Ingredients:

- 1 pound extra-firm tofu, drained and sliced
- 2 tablespoons olive oil
- 1 cup almond meal
- 1 tablespoons yeast
- ½ teaspoon onion powder
- ½ teaspoon garlic powder
- ½ teaspoon oregano

How To:

1. Add all ingredients except tofu and olive oil in a shallow bowl.
2. Mix well.
3. Preheat your oven to 400 degrees F.
4. In a wide bowl, add the almond meal and mix well.
5. Brush tofu with olive oil, dip into the mix and coat well.
6. Line a baking sheet with parchment paper.
7. Transfer coated tofu to the baking sheet.
8. Bake for 20-30 minutes, making sure to flip once until golden brown.
9. Serve and enjoy!

Nutrition (Per Serving)

- Calories: 282
- Fat: 20g
- Carbohydrates: 9g
- Protein: 12g

Hearty Pumpkin Oats

Serving: 3
Prep Time: 5 minutes
Cook Time: 8 minutes
Ingredients:

- 1 cup quick-cooking rolled oats
- ¾ cup almond milk
- ½ cup canned pumpkin puree
- ¼ teaspoon pumpkin pie spice
- 1 teaspoon ground cinnamon

How To:

1. Take a safe microwave bowl and add oats, almond milk, and microwave on high for 1-2 minutes.
2. Add more almond milk if needed to achieve your desired consistency.
3. Cook for 30 seconds more.
4. Stir in pumpkin puree, pumpkin pie spice, ground cinnamon.
5. Heat gently and enjoy!

Nutrition (Per Serving)

- Calories: 229
- Fat: 4g
- Carbohydrates: 38g
- Protein:10g

Wholesome Pumpkin Pie Oatmeal

Serving: 2
Prep Time: 10 minutes
Cook Time: 10 minutes
Smart Points: 6
Ingredients:

- ½ cup canned pumpkin, low sodium
- Mashed banana as needed
- ¾ cup unsweetened almond milk
- ½ teaspoon pumpkin pie spice
- 1 cup oats

How To:

1. Mash banana using a fork and mix in the remaining ingredients (except oats) and mix well.
2. Add oats and finely stir.
3. Transfer mixture to a pot and let the oats cook until it has absorbed the liquid and is tender.
4. Serve and enjoy!

Nutrition (Per Serving)

- Calories: 264
- Fat: 4g
- Carbohydrates: 52g
- Protein: 7g

Power-Packed Oatmeal

Serving: 2
Prep Time: 10-15 minutes
Cook Time: 5 minutes
Ingredients:

- ¼ cup quick-cooking oats
- ¼ cup almond milk
- 2 tablespoons low fat Greek yogurt
- ¼ banana, mashed
- 2-1/4 tablespoons flaxseed meal

How To:

1. Whisk in all of the ingredients in a bowl.
2. Transfer the bowl to your fridge and let it refrigerate for 15 minutes.
3. Serve and enjoy!

Nutrition (Per Serving)

- Calories:
- Fat: 11g
- Carbohydrates: 27g
- Protein: 10g

Chia Porridge

Serving: 2
Prep Time: 10 minutes
Cook Time: 5-10 minutes
Ingredients:

- 1 tablespoon chia seeds
- 1 tablespoon ground flaxseed
- 1/3 cup coconut cream
- ½ cup water
- 1 teaspoon vanilla extract
- 1 tablespoon almond butter

How To:

1. Add chia seeds, coconut cream, flaxseed, water and vanilla to a small pot.
2. Stir and let it sit for 5 minutes.
3. Add almond butter and place pot over low heat.
4. Keep stirring as almond butter melts.
5. Once the porridge is hot/not boiling, pour into bowl.
6. Enjoy!
7. Add a few berries or a dash of cream for extra flavor.

Nutrition (Per Serving)

- Calories: 410
- Fat: 38g
- Carbohydrates: 10g
- Protein: 6g

Mouthwatering Chicken Porridge

Serving: 4
Prep Time: 1 hour
Cook Time: 10-20 minutes
Ingredients:

- 1 cup jasmine rice
- 1 pound steamed/cooked chicken legs
- 5 cups chicken broth
- 4 cups water
- 1 ½ cups fresh ginger
- Green onions
- Toasted cashew nuts

How To:

1. Place the rice in your fridge and allow it to chill 1 hour prior to cooking.
2. Take the rice out and add it to your Instant Pot.
3. Pour in chicken broth and water.
4. Lock the lid and cook on PORRIDGE mode, using the default settings and parameters.
5. Release the pressure naturally over 10 minutes.
6. Open the lid.
7. Remove the meat from the chicken legs and add the meat to your soup.
8. Stir well over Sauté mode.
9. Season with a bit of flavored vinegar and enjoy with a garnish of nuts and onion.

Nutrition (Per Serving)

- Calories: 206
- Fat: 8g
- Carbohydrates: 8g
- Protein: 23g

Simple Blueberry Oatmeal

Serving: 4
Prep Time: 10 minutes
Cooking Time: 8 hours
Ingredients:

- 1 cup blueberries
- 1 cup steel-cut oats
- 1 cup coconut milk
- 2 tablespoons agave nectar
- ½ teaspoon vanilla extract
- Coconut flakes, garnish

How To:

1. Grease Slow Cooker with cooking spray.
2. Add oats, milk, nectar, blueberries, and vanilla.
3. Toss well.
4. Place lid and cook on LOW for 8 hours.
5. Divide between serving bowls and serve.
6. Enjoy!

Nutrition (Per Serving)

- Calories: 202
- Fat: 6g
- Carbohydrates: 12g
- Protein: 6g

The Decisive Apple "Porridge"

Serving: 2
Prep Time: 10 minutes
Cook Time: 5 minutes
Ingredients:

- 1 large apple, peeled, cored and grated
- 1 cup unsweetened almond milk
- 1 ½ tablespoons sunflower seeds
- 1/8 cup fresh blueberries
- ¼ teaspoon fresh vanilla bean extract

How To:

1. Take a large pan and add sunflower seeds, vanilla extract, almond milk, apples, and stir.
2. Place over medium-low heat.
3. Cook for 5 minutes, making sure to keep the mixture stirring.
4. Transfer to a serving bowl.
5. Serve and enjoy!

Nutrition (Per Serving)

- Calories: 123
- Fat: 1.3g
- Carbohydrates:23g
- Protein: 4g

The Unique Smoothie Bowl

Serving: 2
Prep Time: 10 minutes
Cook Time: Nil
Ingredients:

- 2 cups baby spinach leaves
- 1 cup coconut almond milk
- ¼ cup low fat cream
- 2 tablespoons flaxseed oil
- 2 tablespoons chia seeds
- 2 tablespoons walnuts, roughly chopped
- A handful of fresh berries

How To:

1. Add spinach leaves, coconut almond milk, cream and flaxseed oil to a blender.
2. Blitz until smooth.
3. Pour smoothie into serving bowls.
4. Sprinkle chia seeds, berries, walnuts on top.
5. Serve and enjoy!

Nutrition (Per Serving)

- Calories: 380
- Fat: 36g
- Carbohydrates: 12g
- Protein: 5g

Cinnamon and Coconut Porridge

Serving: 4
Prep Time: 5 minutes
Cook Time:5 minutes
Ingredients:

- 2 cups water
- 1 cup coconut cream
- ½ cup unsweetened dried coconut, shredded
- 2 tablespoons flaxseed meal
- 1 tablespoon almond butter
- 1 ½ teaspoons stevia
- 1 teaspoon cinnamon
- Toppings as blueberries

How To:

1. Add the listed ingredients to a small pot, mix well.
2. Transfer pot to stove and place over medium-low heat.
3. Bring to mix to a slow boil.
4. Stir well and remove from the heat.
5. Divide the mix into equal servings and let them sit for 10 minutes.
6. Top with your desired toppings and enjoy!

Nutrition (Per Serving)

- Calories: 171
- Fat: 16g
- Carbohydrates: 6g
- Protein: 2g

Morning Porridge

Serving: 2
Prep Time: 15 minutes
Cook Time: Nil
Ingredients:

- 2 tablespoons coconut flour
- 2 tablespoons vanilla protein powder
- 3 tablespoons Golden Flaxseed meal
- 1 ½ cups almond milk, unsweetened
- Powdered erythritol

How To:

1. Take a bowl and mix in flaxseed meal, protein powder, coconut flour and mix well.
2. Add mix to the saucepan (place over medium heat).
3. Add almond milk and stir, let the mixture thicken .
4. Add your desired amount of sweetener and serve.
5. Enjoy!

Nutrition (Per Serving)

- Calories: 259
- Fat: 13g
- Carbohydrates: 5g
- Protein: 16g

Vanilla Sweet Potato Porridge

Serving: 5
Prep Time: 10 minutes
Cook Time: 8 hours
Ingredients:

- 6 sweet potatoes, peeled and cut into 1-inch cubes
- 1 ½ cups light coconut milk
- 1 teaspoon ground cinnamon
- 1 teaspoon ground cardamom
- 1 teaspoon pure vanilla extract
- 1 cup raisins
- Pinch of salt

How To:

1. Add sweet potatoes coconut milk, vanilla, cardamom, cinnamon to your Slow Cooker.
2. Close lid and cook on LOW for 8 hours.
3. Open the lid and mash the whole mixture using potato masher to mash the sweet potatoes, stir well.
4. Stir in raisins, salt and serve.
5. Serve and enjoy!

Nutrition (Per Serving)

- Calories: 317
- Fat: 4g
-
- Carbohydrates: 71g
- Protein: 4g

A Nice German Oatmeal

Serving: 3
Prep Time: 10 minutes
Cook Time: 8 hours
Ingredients:

- 1 cup steel-cut oats
- 3 cups water
- 6 ounces coconut milk
- 2 tablespoons cocoa powder
- 1 tablespoon brown sugar
- 1 tablespoon coconut, shredded

How to
1. Grease the Slow Cooker well.
2. Add the listed ingredients to your Cooker and stir.
3. Place lid and cook on LOW for 8 hours.
4. Divide amongst serving bowls and enjoy!

Nutrition (Per Serving)

- Calories: 200
- Fat: 4g
-
- Carbohydrates: 11g
- Protein: 5g

Very Nutty Banana Oatmeal

Serving: 4
Prep Time: 15 minutes
Cook Time: 7-9 hours
Ingredients:

- 1 cup steel-cut oats
- 1 ripe banana, mashed
- 2 cups unsweetened almond milk
- 1 cup water
- 1 ½ tablespoons honey
- ½ teaspoon vanilla extract
- ¼ cup almonds, chopped
- 1 teaspoon ground cinnamon
- ¼ teaspoon ground nutmeg

How To:
1. Grease the Slow Cooker well.
2. Add the listed ingredients to your Slow Cooker and stir.
3. Cover with lid and cook on LOW for 7-9 hours.
4. Serve and enjoy!

Nutrition (Per Serving)

- Calories: 230
- Fat: 7g
- Carbohydrates: 40g
- Protein: 5g

Cool Coconut Flatbread

Serving: 4
Prep Time: 15 minutes
Cooking Time: 10 minutes
Ingredients:

- 1 ½ tablespoons coconut flour
- ¼ teaspoon baking powder
- 1/8 teaspoon sunflower seeds
- 1 tablespoon coconut oil, melted
- 1 whole egg

How To:
1. Preheat your oven to 350 degrees F.
2. Add coconut flour, baking powder, sunflower seeds.
3. Add coconut oil, eggs and stir well until mixed.
4. Leave the batter for several minutes.
5. Pour half the batter onto the baking pan.
6. Spread it to form a circle, repeat with remaining batter.
7. Bake in the oven for 10 minutes.
8. Once you get a golden brown texture, let it cool and serve.
9. Enjoy!

Nutrition (Per Serving)

- Total Carbs: 9 (%)
- Fiber: 3g
-
- Protein: 8g (%)
- Fat: 20g (%)

Perfect Homemade Pickled Ginger Gari

Serving: 8
Prep Time: 40 minute
Cook Time: 5 minutes
Ingredients:

- About 8 ounces of fresh ginger root, completely peeled
- 1 teaspoon and extra ½ teaspoon of fine sunflower seeds
- 1 cup vinegar, rice
- 1/3 cup sugar, white

How To:
1. Cut your ginger into small-sized chunks and transfer them to a bowl.
2. Season with sunflower seeds and stir, let the mixture sit for at least 30 minutes.
3. Take a saucepan and add sugar and vinegar, heat it up, bring the mixture to a boil and keep boiling until the sugar has completely dissolved.
4. Pour the liquid over your ginger pieces.
5. Let it cool and wait until the water changes color.
6. Enjoy!
7. Alternatively, store in jars and use as needed.

Nutrition (Per Serving)

- Calories: 14
- Fat: 0.1g
- Carbohydrates: 3g
- Protein: 0.1g

Avocado and Blueberry Medley

Serving: 4
Prep Time: 5 minutes
Cook Time: Nil
Ingredients:

- 1 frozen banana
- 2 avocados, quartered
- 2 cups berries
- Maple syrup as needed

How To:

1. Take your blender and add all ingredients except maple syrup.
2. Add ice water and blend.
3. Garnish with syrup and pour in smoothie glasses.
4. Enjoy!

Nutrition (Per Serving)

- Calories: 250
- Fat: 13g
- Carbohydrates: 40g
- Protein 4g

Healthy Zucchini Stir Fry

Serving: 4
Prep Time: 10 minutes
Cook Time: 10 minutes
Ingredients:

- 2 heaped tablespoons olive oil
- 1 medium-sized onion, sliced thinly
- 2 medium-sized zucchini, cut up into thin sized strips
- 2 heaped tablespoons teriyaki flavored sauce, low sodium
- 1 tablespoon coconut aminos
- 1 tablespoon sesame seed, toasted
- Ground pepper (black) as much as needed

How To:

1. Take a skillet and place it over medium level heat.
2. Add onions, and stir-cook for 5 minutes.
3. Add your zucchini and stir-cook for 1 minute more.
4. Gently add the sauces alongside the sesame seeds.
5. Cook for 5 minutes more until the zucchini are soft.
6. Finally, add the pepper and enjoy!

Nutrition (Per Serving)

- Calories: 110
- Fat: 9g
- Carbohydrates: 8g
- Protein: 3g

Herbed Parmesan Walnuts

Serving: 4
Prep Time: 5 minutes
Cook Time: 30 minutes
Ingredients:

- ½ cup kite ricotta/cashew cheese
- ½ teaspoon Italian herb seasoning and garlic sunflower seeds
- 1 teaspoon parsley flakes
- 2 cups walnuts
- 1 egg white

How To:

1. Preheat your oven to 250 degrees F.
2. Take a bowl and add all ingredients except the egg white and walnuts.
3. Whisk in the egg white, stir in halved walnuts and mix well.
4. Transfer the mixture to a greased baking sheet and bake for 30 minutes.
5. Serve and enjoy!

Nutrition (Per Serving)

- Calories: 220
- Fat: 21g
- Carbohydrates: 4g
- Protein 8g

Amazing Scrambled Turkey Eggs

Serving: 2
Prep Time: 15 minutes
Cook Time: 15 minutes
Ingredients:

- 1 tablespoon coconut oil
- 1 medium red bell pepper, diced
- ½ medium yellow onion, diced
- ¼ teaspoon hot pepper sauce
- 3 large free-range eggs
- ¼ teaspoon black pepper, freshly ground
- ¼ teaspoon salt

How To:

1. Set a pan to medium-high heat, add coconut oil, let it heat up.
2. Add onions and sauté.
3. Add turkey and red pepper .
4. Cook until the turkey is cooked.
5. Take a bowl and beat eggs, stir in salt and pepper.
6. Pour eggs in the pan with turkey and gently cook and scramble eggs.
7. Top with hot sauce and enjoy!

Nutrition (Per Serving)

- Calories: 435
- Fat: 30g
- Carbohydrates: 34g
- Protein: 16g

Egg and Bacon Cups

Serving: 6
Prep Time: 10 minutes
Cook Time: 15 minutes
Ingredients:

- 2 bacon strips
- 2 large eggs
- A handful of fresh spinach
- ¼ cup cheese
- Salt and pepper to taste

How To:

1. Preheat your oven to 400 degrees F.
2. Fry bacon in a skillet over medium heat, drain the oil and keep them on the side.
3. Take muffin tin and grease with oil.
4. Line with a slice of bacon, press down the bacon well, making sure that the ends are sticking out (to be used as handles).
5. Take a bowl and beat eggs.
6. Drain and pat the spinach dry.
7. Add the spinach to the eggs.
8. Add a quarter of the mixture in each of your muffin tins.
9. Sprinkle cheese and season.
10. Bake for 15 minutes.
11. Enjoy!

Nutrition (Per Serving)

- Calories: 101
- Fat: 7g
- Carbohydrates: 2g
- Protein: 8g
- Fiber: 1g
- Net Carbs: 1g

Pepperoni Omelet

Serving: 2
Prep Time: 5 minutes
Cook Time: 20 minutes
Ingredients:

- 3 eggs
- 7 pepperoni slices
- 1 teaspoon coconut cream
- Salt and freshly ground black pepper, to taste
- 1 tablespoons butter

How To:

1. Take a bowl and whisk eggs with all the remaining ingredients in it.
2. Then take a skillet and heat the butter.
3. Pour ¼ of the egg mixture into your skillet.
4. After that, cook for 2 minutes per side.
5. Repeat to use the entire batter.
6. Serve warm and enjoy!

Nutrition (Per Serving)

- Calories: 141
- Fat: 11.5g
- Carbohydrates: 0.6g
- Protein: 8.9g

Cinnamon Baked Apple Chips

Serving: 2
Prep Time: 5 minutes
Cook Time: 2 hours
Ingredients:

- 1 teaspoon cinnamon
- 1-2 apples

How To:

1. Preheat your oven to 200 degrees F.
2. Take a sharp knife and slice apples into thin slices.
3. Discard seeds.
4. Line a baking sheet with parchment paper and arrange apples on it.
5. Make sure they do not overlap.
6. Once done, sprinkle cinnamon over apples.
7. Bake in the oven for 1 hour.
8. Flip and bake for an hour more until no longer moist.
9. Serve and enjoy!

Nutrition (Per Serving)

- Calories: 147
- Fat: 0g
- Carbohydrates: 39g
- Protein: 1g

Herb and Avocado Omelet

Serving: 2
Prep Time: 2 minutes
Cook Time: 10 minutes
Ingredients:

- 3 large free-range eggs
- ½ medium avocado, sliced
- ½ cup almonds, sliced
- Salt and pepper as needed

How To:

1. Take a non-stick skillet and place it over medium-high heat.
2. Take a bowl and add eggs, beat the eggs.
3. Pour into the skillet and cook for 1 minute.
4. Reduce heat to low and cook for 4 minutes.
5. Top the omelet with almonds and avocado.
6. Sprinkle salt and pepper and serve.
7. Enjoy!

Nutrition (Per Serving)

- Calories: 193
- Fat: 15g
- Carbohydrates: 5g
- Protein: 10g

Classic Apple and Cinnamon Oatmeal

Serving: 4
Prep Time: 15 minutes
Cook Time: 7-9 hours
Ingredients:

- 1 apple, cored, peeled and diced
- 1 cup steel-cut oats
- 2 ½ cups unsweetened vanilla almond milk
- 2 tablespoons honey
- ½ teaspoon vanilla extract
- 1 teaspoon ground cinnamon

How To:
1. Grease the Slow Cooker well.
2. Add the listed ingredients to your Slow Cooker and stir.
3. Cover with lid and cook on LOW for 7-9 hours.
4. Serve and enjoy!

Nutrition (Per Serving)

- Calories: 126
- Fat: 3g
- Carbohydrates: 25g
- Protein: 3g

Carrot and Zucchini Oatmeal

Serving: 3
Prep Time: 10 minutes
Cook Time: 8 hours
Ingredients:

- ½ cup steel cut oats
- 1 cup coconut milk
- 1 carrot, grated
- ¼ zucchini, grated
- Pinch of nutmeg
- ½ teaspoon cinnamon powder
- 2 tablespoons brown sugar
- ¼ cup pecans, chopped

How To:
1. Grease the Slow Cooker well.
2. Add oats, zucchini, milk, carrot, nutmeg, cloves, sugar, cinnamon and stir well.
3. Place lid and cook on LOW for 8 hours.
4. Divide amongst serving bowls and enjoy!

Nutrition (Per Serving)

- Calories: 200
- Fat: 4g
- Carbohydrates: 11g
- Protein: 5g

Blueberry and Walnut "Steel" Oatmeal

Serving: 8
Prep Time: 5 minutes
Cook Time: 7-8 hours
Ingredients:

- 2 cups steel-cut oats
- 6 cups water
- 2 cups low-fat milk
- 2 cups fresh blueberries
- 1 ripe banana, mashed
- 1 teaspoon vanilla extract
- 2 teaspoons ground cinnamon
- 2 tablespoons brown sugar
- Pinch of salt
- ½ cup walnuts, chopped

How To:
1. Grease the inside of your Slow Cooker.
2. Add oats, milk, water, blueberries, banana, vanilla, brown sugar, cinnamon and salt to your Slow Cooker.
3. Stir.
4. Place lid and cook on LOW for 7-8 hours.
5. Serve warm with a garnish of chopped walnuts.
6. Enjoy!

Nutrition (Per Serving)

- Calories: 372
- Fat: 14g
- Carbohydrates: 56g
- Protein: 8g

Shrimp and Egg Medley

Serving: 4
Prep Time: 15 minutes
Cook Time: nil
Ingredients:

- 4 hard boiled eggs, peeled and chopped
- 1 pound cooked shrimp, peeled and de-veined, chopped
- 1 sprig fresh dill, chopped
- ¼ cup mayonnaise
- 1 teaspoon Dijon mustard
- 4 fresh lettuce leaves

How To:
1. Take a large serving bowl and add the listed ingredients (except lettuce.)
2. Stir well.
3. Serve over bet of lettuce leaves.
4. Enjoy!

Nutrition (Per Serving)

- Calories: 292
- Fat: 17g
- Carbohydrates: 1.6g
- Protein: 30g

Crispy Walnut Crumbles

Serving: 10
Prep Time: 10 minutes
Cook Time: 8 minutes
Ingredients:

- 6 ounces kite ricotta/cashew cheese, grated
- 2 tablespoons walnuts, chopped
- 1 tablespoon almond butter
- ½ tablespoon fresh thyme chopped

How To:

1. Preheat your oven to 350 degrees F.
2. Take two large rimmed baking sheets and line with parchment.
3. Add cheese, almond butter to a food processor and blend.
4. Add walnuts to the mix and pulse.
5. Take a tablespoon and scoop mix onto a baking sheet.
6. Top them with chopped thymes.
7. Bake for 8 minutes, transfer to a cooling rack.
8. Let it cool for 30 minutes.
9. Serve and enjoy!

Nutrition (Per Serving)

- Calories: 80
- Fat: 3g
- Carbohydrates: 7g
- Protein: 7g

Cheesy Zucchini Omelette

Serving: 3
Prep Time: 10 minutes
Cook Time: 20 minutes
Ingredients:

- 4 large eggs
- 2-3 medium zucchinis
- 1-2 garlic cloves, crushed
- 4 tablespoons grated cheese
- Season as needed

How To:

1. Take a bowl and add grated zucchinis, make sure to peel them as the skin is bitter.
2. Take a bowl and break in the eggs, crushed garlic and cheese.
3. Pour the mixture in a hot frying pan with a little bit of oil and place it over medium heat, keep a lid on.
4. Once the egg is cooked nicely, and the bottom is crispy and golden, serve and enjoy with a garnish of chopped parsley.
5. Enjoy!

Nutrition (Per Serving)

- Calories: 289
- Fat: 20g
- Carbohydrates: 7g
- Protein: 21g

Old Fashioned Breakfast Oatmeal

Serving: 4
Prep Time: 10 minutes
Cook Time: 5 minutes
Ingredients:

- 2 ½ cups water
- 1 cup old fashioned oats
- 1 cup apple, peeled, cored and chopped
- 3 tablespoons low-fat butter
- 2 tablespoons palm sugar
- ½ teaspoon cinnamon powder

How To:

1. Add water, oats, apple, butter, cinnamon, and sugar to an Instant Pot.
2. Toss well and lock the lid.
3. Cook on HIGH pressure for 5 minutes.
4. Release the pressure naturally over 10 minutes.
5. Stir oats and divide into bowls.
6. Enjoy!

Nutrition (Per Serving)

- Calories: 191
- Fat: 2g
- Carbohydrates: 9g
- Protein: 5g

Healthy Peach Oatmeal

Serving: 8
Prep Time: 10 minutes
Cook Time: 10 minutes
Ingredients:

- 4 cups old fashioned rolled oats
- 3 ½ cups low-fat milk
- 3 ½ cups water
- 1 teaspoon cinnamon powder
- 1/3 cup palm sugar
- 4 peaches, chopped

How To:

1. Add oats, milk, cinnamon, water, sugar, and peaches to your Instant Pot.
2. Toss well.
3. Lock the lid and cook for 10 minutes on HIGH pressure.
4. Release the pressure naturally over 10 minutes .
5. Divide the mix in bowls and serve!

Nutrition (Per Serving)

- Calories: 192
- Fat: 3g
- Carbohydrates: 12g
- Protein: 4g

Fancy Banana Oatmeal

Serving: 4
Prep Time: 10 minutes
Cook Time: 10 minutes
Ingredients:

- 2 cups water
- 1 cup steel-cut oats
- 1 cup almond milk
- ¼ cup walnuts, chopped
- 2 tablespoons flaxseeds, ground
- 2 tablespoons chia seeds
- 2 bananas, peeled and mashed
- 1 teaspoon vanilla extract
- 1 teaspoon cinnamon powder

How To:

1. Add water, oats, almond milk, flaxseed, walnuts, chia seeds, vanilla, bananas, cinnamon to your Instant Pot and give it a nice toss.
2. Lock the lid and cook on HIGH pressure for 10 minutes.
3. Release the pressure naturally and open the lid.
4. Divide the mix amongst bowls and serve.
5. Enjoy!

Nutrition (Per Serving)

- Calories: 200
- Fat: 4g
- Carbohydrates: 11g
- Protein: 4g

Traditional Frittata

Serving: 6
Prep Time: 10 minutes
Cook Time: 5 minutes
Ingredients:

- 2 tablespoons almond milk
- Just a pinch pepper
- 6 eggs, cracked and whisked
- 2 tablespoons parsley, chopped
- 1 tablespoon low-fat cheese, shredded
- 1 cup of water

How To:

1. Take a bowl and add the eggs, almond milk, pepper, cheese, and parsley. Whisk well.
2. Take a pan that would fit in your Instant Pot and grease with cooking spray.
3. Pour the egg mix into the pan.
4. Add a cup of water to your pot and place a steamer basket.
5. Add the pan in the basket.
6. Lock the lid and cook on HIGH pressure for 5 minutes.
7. Release the pressure naturally over 10 minutes.
8. Remove the lid and divide the frittata amongst serving plates.
9. Enjoy!

Nutrition (Per Serving)

- Calories: 200
- Fat: 4g
- Carbohydrates: 17g
- Protein: 6g

Pepperoni Omelet

Serving: 2
Prep Time: 5 minutes
Cook Time: 20 minutes
Ingredients:

- 3 eggs
- 7 pepperoni slices
- 1 teaspoon coconut cream
- Salt and freshly ground black pepper, to taste
- 1 tablespoon butter

How To:

1. Take a bowl and whisk eggs with all the remaining ingredients in it.
2. Then take a skillet and heat butter.
3. Pour quarter of the egg mixture into your skillet.
4. After that, cook for 2 minutes per side.
5. Repeat to use the entire batter.
6. Serve warm and enjoy!

Nutrition (Per Serving)

- Calories: 141
- Fat: 11.5g
- Carbohydrates: 0.6g
- Protein: 8.9g

Eggy Tomato Scramble

Serving: 2
Prep Time: 10 minutes
Cook Time: 5 minutes
Ingredients:

- 2 whole eggs
- ½ cup fresh basil, chopped
- 2 tablespoons olive oil
- ½ teaspoon red pepper flakes, crushed
- 1 cup grape tomatoes, chopped
- Salt and pepper to taste

How To:

1. Take a bowl and whisk in eggs, salt, pepper, red pepper flakes and mix well.
2. Add tomatoes, basil, and mix.
3. Take a skillet and place over medium-high heat.
4. Add the egg mixture and cook for 5 minutes until cooked and scrambled.
5. Enjoy!

Nutrition (Per Serving)

- Calories: 130
- Fat: 10g
- Carbohydrates: 8g
- Protein: 1.8g

Chapter 2: Lunch Recipes

Fascinating Spinach and Beef Meatballs

Serving: 4
Prep Time: 10 minutes
Cook Time: 20
Ingredients:

- ½ cup onion
- 4 garlic cloves
- 1 whole egg
- ¼ teaspoon oregano
- Pepper as needed
- 1 pound lean ground beef
- 10 ounces spinach

How To:

1. Preheat your oven to 375 degrees F.
2. Take a bowl and mix in the rest of the ingredients, and using your hands, roll into meatballs.
3. Transfer to a sheet tray and bake for 20 minutes.
4. Enjoy!

Nutrition (Per Serving)

- Calorie: 200
- Fat: 8g
- Carbohydrates: 5g
- Protein: 29g

Juicy and Peppery Tenderloin

Serving: 4
Prep Time: 10 minutes
Cook Time: 20
Ingredients:

- 2 teaspoons sage, chopped
- Sunflower seeds and pepper
- 2 1/2 pounds beef tenderloin
- 2 teaspoons thyme, chopped
- 2 garlic cloves, sliced
- 2 teaspoons rosemary, chopped
- 4 teaspoons olive oil

How To:

1. Preheat your oven to 425 degrees F.
2. Take a small knife and cut incisions in the tenderloin; insert one slice of garlic into the incision.
3. Rub meat with oil.
4. Take a bowl and add sunflower seeds, sage, thyme, rosemary, pepper and mix well.
5. Rub the spice mix over tenderloin.
6. Put rubbed tenderloin into the roasting pan and bake for 10 minutes.
7. Lower temperature to 350 degrees F and cook for 20 minutes more until an internal thermometer reads 145 degrees F.
8. Transfer tenderloin to a cutting board and let sit for 15 minutes; slice into 20 pieces and enjoy!

Nutrition (Per Serving)

- Calorie: 183
- Fat: 9g
- Carbohydrates: 1g
- Protein: 24g

Healthy Avocado Beef Patties

Serving: 2
Prep Time: 15 minutes
Cook Time: 10 minutes
Ingredients:

- 1 pound 85% lean ground beef
- 1 small avocado, pitted and peeled
- Fresh ground black pepper as needed

How To:

1. Pre-heat and prepare your broiler to high.
2. Divide beef into two equal-sized patties.
3. Season the patties with pepper accordingly.
4. Broil the patties for 5 minutes per side.
5. Transfer the patties to a platter.
6. Slice avocado into strips and place them on top of the patties.
7. Serve and enjoy!

Nutrition (Per Serving)

- Calories: 568
- Fat: 43g
- Net Carbohydrates: 9g
- Protein: 38g

Ravaging Beef Pot Roast

Serving: 4
Prep Time: 10 minutes
Cook Time: 75 minutes
Ingredients:

- 3 ½ pounds beef roast
- 4 ounces mushrooms, sliced
- 12 ounces beef stock
- 1-ounce onion soup mix
- ½ cup Italian dressing, low sodium, and low fat

How To:

1. Take a bowl and add the stock, onion soup mix and Italian dressing.
2. Stir.
3. Put beef roast in pan.
4. Add mushrooms, stock mix to the pan and cover with foil.
5. Preheat your oven to 300 degrees F.
6. Bake for 1 hour and 15 minutes.
7. Let the roast cool.
8. Slice and serve.
9. Enjoy with the gravy on top!

Nutrition (Per Serving)

- Calories: 700
- Fat: 56g
- Carbohydrates: 10g
- Protein: 70g

Lovely Faux Mac and Cheese

Serving: 4
Prep Time: 15 minutes
Cook Time: 45 minutes
Ingredients:

- 5 cups cauliflower florets
- Sunflower seeds and pepper to taste
- 1 cup coconut almond milk
- ½ cup vegetable broth
- 2 tablespoons coconut flour, sifted
- 1 organic egg, beaten
- 1 cup cashew cheese

How To:

1. Preheat your oven to 350 degrees F.
2. Season florets with sunflower seeds and steam until firm.
3. Place florets in a greased ovenproof dish.
4. Heat coconut almond milk over medium heat in a skillet, make sure to season the oil with sunflower seeds and pepper.
5. Stir in broth and add coconut flour to the mix, stir.
6. Cook until the sauce begins to bubble.
7. Remove heat and add beaten egg.
8. Pour the thick sauce over the cauliflower and mix in cheese.
9. Bake for 30-45 minutes.
10. Serve and enjoy!

Nutrition (Per Serving)

- Calories: 229
- Fat: 14g
- Carbohydrates: 9g
- Protein: 15g

Epic Mango Chicken

Serving: 4
Prep Time: 25 minutes
Cook Time: 10 minutes
Ingredients:

- 2 medium mangoes, peeled and sliced
- 10-ounce coconut almond milk
- 4 teaspoons vegetable oil
- 4 teaspoons spicy curry paste
- 14-ounce chicken breast halves, skinless and boneless, cut in cubes
- 4 medium shallots
- 1 large English cucumber, sliced and seeded

How To:

1. Slice half of the mangoes and add the halves to a bowl.
2. Add mangoes and coconut almond milk to a blender and blend until you have a smooth puree.
3. Keep the mixture on the side.
4. Take a large-sized pot and place it over medium heat, add oil and allow the oil to heat up.
5. Add curry paste and cook for 1 minute until you have a nice fragrance, add shallots and chicken to the pot and cook for 5 minutes.
6. Pour mango puree in to the mix and allow it to heat up.
7. Serve the cooked chicken with mango puree and cucumbers.
8. Enjoy!

Nutrition (Per Serving)

- Calories: 398
- Fat: 20g
- Carbohydrates: 32g
- Protein: 26g

Chicken and Cabbage Platter

Serving: 2
Prep Time: 9 minute
Cook Time: 14 minutes
Ingredients:

- ½ cup sliced onion
- 1 tablespoon sesame garlic-flavored oil
- 2 cups shredded Bok-Choy
- 1/2 cups fresh bean sprouts
- 1 1/2 stalks celery, chopped
- 1 ½ teaspoons minced garlic
- 1/2 teaspoon stevia
- 1/2 cup chicken broth
- 1 tablespoon coconut aminos
- 1/2 tablespoon freshly minced ginger
- 1/2 teaspoon arrowroot
- 2 boneless chicken breasts, cooked and sliced thinly

How To:

1. Shred the cabbage with a knife.
2. Slice onion and add to your platter alongside the rotisserie chicken.
3. Add a dollop of mayonnaise on top and drizzle olive oil over the cabbage.
4. Season with sunflower seeds and pepper according to your taste.
5. Enjoy!

Nutrition (Per Serving)

- Calories: 368
- Fat: 18g
- Net Carbohydrates: 8g
- Protein: 42g
- Fiber: 3g
- Carbohydrates: 11g

Hearty Chicken Liver Stew

Serving: 2
Prep Time: 10 minutes
Cook Time: Nil
Ingredients:

- 10 ounces chicken livers
- 1-ounce onion, chopped
- 2 ounces sour cream
- 1 tablespoon olive oil
- Sunflower seeds to taste

How To:

1. Take a pan and place it over medium heat.
2. Add oil and let it heat up.
3. Add onions and fry until just browned.
4. Add livers and season with sunflower seeds.
5. Cook until livers are half cooked.
6. Transfer the mix to a stew pot.
7. Add sour cream and cook for 20 minutes.
8. Serve and enjoy!

Nutrition (Per Serving)

- Calories: 146
- Fat: 9g
- Carbohydrates: 2g
- Protein: 15g

Chicken Quesadilla

Serving: 2
Prep Time: 10 minutes
Cook Time: 35 minutes
Ingredients:

- ¼ cup ranch dressing
- ½ cup cheddar cheese, shredded
- 20 slices bacon, center-cut
- 2 cups grilled chicken, sliced

How To:

1. Re-heat your oven to 400 degrees F.
2. Line baking sheet using parchment paper.
3. Weave bacon into two rectangles and bake for 30 minutes.
4. Lay grilled chicken over bacon square, drizzling ranch dressing on top.
5. Sprinkle cheddar cheese and top with another bacon square.
6. Bake for 5 minutes more.
7. Slice and serve.
8. Enjoy!

Nutrition (Per Serving)

- Calories: 619
- Fat: 35g
- Carbohydrates: 2g
- Protein: 79g

Mustard Chicken

Serving: 2
Prep Time: 10 minutes
Cook Time: 40 minutes
Ingredients:

- 2 chicken breasts
- 1/4 cup chicken broth
- 2 tablespoons mustard
- 1 1/2 tablespoons olive oil
- 1/2 teaspoon paprika
- 1/2 teaspoon chili powder
- 1/2 teaspoon garlic powder

How To:

1. Take a small bowl and mix mustard, olive oil, paprika, chicken broth, garlic powder, chicken broth, and chili.
2. Add chicken breast and marinate for 30 minutes.
3. Take a lined baking sheet and arrange the chicken.
4. Bake for 35 minutes at 375 degrees F.
5. Serve and enjoy!

Nutrition (Per Serving)

- Calories: 531
- Fat: 23g
- Carbohydrates: 10g
- Protein: 64g

Chicken and Carrot Stew

Serving: 4
Prep Time: 15 minutes
Cook Time: 6 hours
Ingredients:

- 4 boneless chicken breast, cubed
- 3 cups of carrots, peeled and cubed
- 1 cup onion, chopped
- 1 cup tomatoes, chopped
- 1 teaspoon of dried thyme
- 2 cups of chicken broth
- 2 garlic cloves, minced
- Sunflower seeds and pepper as needed

How To:

1. Add all of the listed ingredients to a Slow Cooker.
2. Stir and close the lid.
3. Cook for 6 hours.
4. Serve hot and enjoy!

Nutrition (Per Serving)

- Calories: 182
- Fat: 3g
- Carbohydrates: 10g
- Protein: 39g

The Delish Turkey Wrap

Serving: 6

Prep Time: 10 minutes

Cook Time: 10 minutes

Ingredients:

- 1 ¼ pounds ground turkey, lean
- 4 green onions, minced
- 1 tablespoon olive oil
- 1 garlic clove, minced
- 2 teaspoons chili paste
- 8-ounce water chestnut, diced
- 3 tablespoons hoisin sauce
- 2 tablespoon coconut aminos
- 1 tablespoon rice vinegar
- 12 almond butter lettuce leaves
- 1/8 teaspoon sunflower seeds

How To:

1. Take a pan and place it over medium heat, add turkey and garlic to the pan.
2. Heat for 6 minutes until cooked.
3. Take a bowl and transfer turkey to the bowl.
4. Add onions and water chestnuts.
5. Stir in hoisin sauce, coconut aminos, vinegar and chili paste.
6. Toss well and transfer mix to lettuce leaves.
7. Serve and enjoy!

Nutrition (Per Serving)

- Calories: 162
- Fat: 4g
- Net Carbohydrates: 7g
- Protein: 23g

Almond butternut Chicken

Serving: 4

Prep Time: 15 minutes

Cook Time: 30 minutes

Ingredients:

- ½ pound Nitrate free bacon
- 6 chicken thighs, boneless and skinless
- 2-3 cups almond butternut squash, cubed
- Extra virgin olive oil
- Fresh chopped sage
- Sunflower seeds and pepper as needed

How To:

1. Prepare your oven by preheating it to 425 degrees F.
2. Take a large skillet and place it over medium-high heat, add bacon and fry until crispy.
3. Take a slice of bacon and place it on the side, crumble the bacon.
4. Add cubed almond butternut squash in the bacon grease and sauté, season with sunflower seeds and pepper.
5. Once the squash is tender, remove skillet and transfer to a plate.
6. Add coconut oil to the skillet and add chicken thighs, cook for 10 minutes.
7. Season with sunflower seeds and pepper.
8. Remove skillet from stove and transfer to oven.
9. Bake for 12-15 minutes, top with the crumbled bacon and sage.
10. Enjoy!

Nutrition (Per Serving)

- Calories: 323
- Fat: 19g
- Carbohydrates: 8g
- Protein: 12g

Zucchini Zoodles with Chicken and Basil

Serving: 3
Prep Time: 10 minutes
Cook Time: 10 minutes
Ingredients:

- 2 chicken fillets, cubed
- 2 tablespoons ghee
- 1 pound tomatoes, diced
- ½ cup basil, chopped
- ¼ cup almond milk
- 1 garlic clove, peeled, minced
- 1 zucchini, shredded

How To:

1. Sauté cubed chicken in ghee until no longer pink.
2. Add tomatoes and season with sunflower seeds.
3. Simmer and reduce liquid.
4. Prepare your zucchini Zoodles by shredding zucchini in a food processor.
5. Add basil, garlic, coconut almond milk to the chicken and cook for a few minutes.
6. Add half of the zucchini Zoodles to a bowl and top with creamy tomato basil chicken.
7. Enjoy!

Nutrition (Per Serving)

- Calories: 540
- Fat: 27g
- Carbohydrates: 13g
- Protein: 59g

Duck with Cucumber and Carrots

Serving: 8
Prep Time: 10 minutes
Cook Time: 40 minutes
Ingredients:

- 1 duck, cut up into medium pieces
- 1 chopped cucumber, chopped
- 1 tablespoon low sodium vegetable stock
- 2 carrots, chopped
- 2 cups of water
- Black pepper as needed
- 1-inch ginger piece, grated

How To:

1. Add duck pieces to your Instant Pot.
2. Add cucumber, stock, carrots, water, ginger, pepper and stir.
3. Lock up the lid and cook on LOW pressure for 40 minutes.
4. Release the pressure naturally.
5. Serve and enjoy!

Nutrition (Per Serving)

- Calories: 206
- Fats: 7g
- Carbs: 28g
- Protein: 16g

Parmesan Baked Chicken

Serving: 2
Prep Time: 5 minutes
Cook Time: 20 minutes
Ingredients:

- 2 tablespoons ghee
- 2 boneless chicken breasts, skinless
- Pink sunflower seeds
- Freshly ground black pepper
- ½ cup mayonnaise, low fat
- ¼ cup parmesan cheese, grated
- 1 tablespoon dried Italian seasoning, low fat, low sodium
- ¼ cup crushed pork rinds

How To:

1. Preheat your oven to 425 degrees F.
2. Take a large baking dish and coat with ghee.
3. Pat chicken breasts dry and wrap with a towel.
4. Season with sunflower seeds and pepper.
5. Place in baking dish.
6. Take a small bowl and add mayonnaise, parmesan cheese, Italian seasoning.
7. Slather mayo mix evenly over chicken breast.
8. Sprinkle crushed pork rinds on top.
9. Bake for 20 minutes until topping is browned.
10. Serve and enjoy!

Nutrition (Per Serving)

- Calories: 850
- Fat: 67g
- Carbohydrates: 2g
- Protein: 60g

Buffalo Chicken Lettuce Wraps

Serving: 2
Prep Time: 35 minutes
Cook Time: 10 minutes
Ingredients:

- 3 chicken breasts, boneless and cubed
- 20 slices of almond butter lettuce leaves
- ¾ cup cherry tomatoes halved
- 1 avocado, chopped
- ¼ cup green onions, diced
- ½ cup ranch dressing
- ¾ cup hot sauce

How To:

1. Take a mixing bowl and add chicken cubes and hot sauce, mix.
2. Place in the fridge and let it marinate for 30 minutes.
3. Preheat your oven to 400 degrees F.
4. Place coated chicken on a cookie pan and bake for 9 minutes.
5. Assemble lettuce serving cups with equal amounts of lettuce, green onions, tomatoes, ranch dressing, and cubed chicken.
6. Serve and enjoy!

Nutrition (Per Serving)

- Calories: 106
- Fat: 6g
- Net Carbohydrates: 2g
- Protein: 5g

Crazy Japanese Potato and Beef Croquettes

Serving: 10
Prep Time: 10 minute
Cook Time: 20 minutes
Ingredients:

- 3 medium russet potatoes, peeled and chopped
- 1 tablespoon almond butter
- 1 tablespoon vegetable oil
- 3 onions, diced
- ¾ pound ground beef
- 4 teaspoons light coconut aminos
- All-purpose flour for coating
- 2 eggs, beaten
- Panko bread crumbs for coating
- ½ cup oil, frying

How To:

1. Take a saucepan and place it over medium-high heat; add potatoes and sunflower seeds water, boil for 16 minutes.
2. Remove water and put potatoes in another bowl, add almond butter and mash the potatoes.
3. Take a frying pan and place it over medium heat, add 1 tablespoon oil and let it heat up.
4. Add onions and stir fry until tender.
5. Add coconut aminos to beef to onions.
6. Keep frying until beef is browned.
7. Mix the beef with the potatoes evenly.
8. Take another frying pan and place it over medium heat; add half a cup of oil.
9. Form croquettes using the mashed potato mixture and coat them with flour, then eggs and finally breadcrumbs.
10. Fry patties until golden on all sides.
11. Enjoy!

Nutrition (Per Serving)

- Calories: 239
- Fat: 4g
- Carbohydrates: 20g
- Protein: 10g

Spicy Chili Crackers

Serving: 30 crackers
Prep Time: 15 minutes
Cooking Time: 60 minutes
Ingredients:

- ¾ cup almond flour
- ¼ cup coconut four
- ¼ cup coconut flour
- ½ teaspoon paprika
- ½ teaspoon cumin
- 1 ½ teaspoons chili pepper spice
- 1 teaspoon onion powder
- ½ teaspoon sunflower seeds
- 1 whole egg
- ¼ cup unsalted almond butter

How To:

1. Preheat your oven to 350 degrees F.
2. Line a baking sheet with parchment paper and keep it on the side.
3. Add ingredients to your food processor and pulse until you have a nice dough.
4. Divide dough into two equal parts.
5. Place one ball on a sheet of parchment paper and cover with another sheet; roll it out.
6. Cut into crackers and repeat with the other ball.
7. Transfer the prepped dough to a baking tray and bake for 8-10 minutes.

8. Remove from oven and serve.

9. Enjoy!

Nutrition (Per Serving)

- Total Carbs: 2.8g
- Fiber: 1g
- Protein: 1.6g
- Fat: 4.1g

Golden Eggplant Fries

Serving: 8

Prep Time: 10 minutes

Cook Time: 15 minutes

Ingredients:

- 2 eggs
- 2 cups almond flour
- 2 tablespoons coconut oil, spray
- 2 eggplant, peeled and cut thinly
- Sunflower seeds and pepper

How To:

1. Preheat your oven to 400 degrees F.

2. Take a bowl and mix with sunflower seeds and black pepper.

3. Take another bowl and beat eggs until frothy.

4. Dip the eggplant pieces into the eggs.

5. Then coat them with the flour mixture.

6. Add another layer of flour and egg.

7. Then, take a baking sheet and grease with coconut oil on top.

8. Bake for about 15 minutes.

9. Serve and enjoy!

Nutrition (Per Serving)

- Calories: 212
- Fat: 15.8g
- Carbohydrates: 12.1g
- Protein: 8.6g

Traditional Black Bean Chili

Serving: 4
Prep Time: 10 minutes
Cooking Time: 4 hours
Ingredients:

- 1 ½ cups red bell pepper, chopped
- 1 cup yellow onion, chopped
- 1 ½ cups mushrooms, sliced
- 1 tablespoon olive oil
- 1 tablespoon chili powder
- 2 garlic cloves, minced
- 1 teaspoon chipotle chili pepper, chopped
- ½ teaspoon cumin, ground
- 16 ounces canned black beans, drained and rinsed
- 2 tablespoons cilantro, chopped
- 1 cup tomatoes, chopped

How To:

1. Add red bell peppers, onion, dill, mushrooms, chili powder, garlic, chili pepper, cumin, black beans, tomatoes to your Slow Cooker.
2. Stir well.
3. Place lid and cook on HIGH for 4 hours.
4. Sprinkle cilantro on top.
5. Serve and enjoy!

Nutrition (Per Serving)

- Calories: 211
- Fat: 3g
- Carbohydrates: 22g
- Protein: 5g

Very Wild Mushroom Pilaf

Serving: 4
Prep Time: 10 minutes
Cooking Time: 3 hours
Ingredients:

- 1 cup wild rice
- 2 garlic cloves, minced
- 6 green onions, chopped
- 2 tablespoons olive oil
- ½ pound baby Bella mushrooms
- 2 cups water

How To:

1. Add rice, garlic, onion, oil, mushrooms and water to your Slow Cooker.
2. Stir well until mixed.
3. Place lid and cook on LOW for 3 hours.
4. Stir pilaf and divide between serving platters.
5. Enjoy!

Nutrition (Per Serving)

- Calories: 210
- Fat: 7g
- Carbohydrates: 16g
- Protein: 4g

Green Palak Paneer

Serving: 4
Prep Time: 5 minutes
Cook Time: 10 minutes
Ingredients:

- 1 pound spinach
- 2 cups cubed paneer (vegan)
- 2 tablespoons coconut oil
- 1 teaspoon cumin
- 1 chopped up onion
- 1-2 teaspoons hot green chili minced up
- 1 teaspoon minced garlic
- 15 cashews
- 4 tablespoons almond milk
- 1 teaspoon Garam masala
- Flavored vinegar as needed

How To:

1. Add cashews and milk to a blender and blend well.
2. Set your pot to Sauté mode and add coconut oil; allow the oil to heat up.
3. Add cumin seeds, garlic, green chilies, ginger and sauté for 1 minute.
4. Add onion and sauté for 2 minutes.
5. Add chopped spinach, flavored vinegar and a cup of water.
6. Lock up the lid and cook on HIGH pressure for 10 minutes.
7. Quick-release the pressure.
8. Add ½ cup of water and blend to a paste.
9. Add cashew paste, paneer and Garam Masala and stir thoroughly.
10. Serve over hot rice!

Nutrition (Per Serving)

- Calories: 367
- Fat: 26g
- Carbohydrates: 21g
- Protein: 16g

Sporty Baby Carrots

Serving: 4
Prep Time: 5 minutes
Cook Time: 5 minutes
Ingredients:

- 1 pound baby carrots
- 1 cup water
- 1 tablespoon clarified ghee
- 1 tablespoon chopped up fresh mint leaves
- Sea flavored vinegar as needed

How To:

1. Place a steamer rack on top of your pot and add the carrots.
2. Add water .
3. Lock the lid and cook at HIGH pressure for 2 minutes.
4. Do a quick release.
5. Pass the carrots through a strainer and drain them.
6. Wipe the insert clean.
7. Return the insert to the pot and set the pot to Sauté mode.

8. Add clarified butter and allow it to melt.

9. Add mint and sauté for 30 seconds.

10. Add carrots to the insert and sauté well.

11. Remove them and sprinkle with bit of flavored vinegar on top.

12. Enjoy!

Nutrition (Per Serving)

- Calories: 131
- Fat: 10g
- Carbohydrates: 11g
- Protein: 1g

Saucy Garlic Greens

Serving: 4
Prep Time: 5 minutes
Cook Time: 20 minutes
Ingredients:

- 1 bunch of leafy greens

Sauce

- ½ cup cashews soaked in water for 10 minutes
- ¼ cup water
- 1 tablespoon lemon juice
- 1 teaspoon coconut aminos
- 1 clove peeled whole clove
- 1/8 teaspoon of flavored vinegar

How To:

1. Make the sauce by draining and discarding the soaking water from your cashews and add the cashews to a blender.

2. Add fresh water, lemon juice, flavored vinegar, coconut aminos, garlic.

3. Blitz until you have a smooth cream and transfer to bowl.

4. Add ½ cup of water to the pot.

5. Place the steamer basket to the pot and add the greens in the basket.

6. Lock the lid and steam for 1 minute.

7. Quick-release the pressure.

8. Transfer the steamed greens to strainer and extract excess water.

9. Place the greens into a mixing bowl.

10. Add lemon garlic sauce and toss.

11. Enjoy!

Nutrition (Per Serving)

- Calories: 77
- Fat: 5g
- Carbohydrates: 0g
- Protein: 2g

Garden Salad
Serving: 6
Prep Time: 5 minutes
Cook Time: 20 minutes
Ingredients:

- 1 pound raw peanuts in shell
- 1 bay leaf
- 2 medium-sized chopped up tomatoes
- ½ cup diced up green pepper
- ½ cup diced up sweet onion

- ¼ cup finely diced hot pepper
- ¼ cup diced up celery
- 2 tablespoons olive oil
- ¾ teaspoon flavored vinegar
- ¼ teaspoon freshly ground black pepper

How To:

1. Boil your peanuts for 1 minute and rinse them.
2. The skin will be soft, so discard the skin.
3. Add 2 cups of water to the Instant Pot.
4. Add bay leaf and peanuts.
5. Lock the lid and cook on HIGH pressure for 20 minutes.
6. Drain the water.
7. Take a large bowl and add the peanuts, diced up vegetables.
8. Whisk in olive oil, lemon juice, pepper in another bowl.
9. Pour the mixture over the salad and mix.
10. Enjoy!

Nutrition (Per Serving)

- Calories: 140
- Fat: 4g

- Carbohydrates: 24g
- Protein: 5g

Spicy Cabbage Dish
Serving: 4
Prep Time: 10 minutes
Cooking Time: 4 hours
Ingredients:

- 2 yellow onions, chopped
- 10 cups red cabbage, shredded
- 1 cup plums, pitted and chopped
- 1 teaspoon cinnamon powder
- 1 garlic clove, minced

- 1 teaspoon cumin seeds
- ¼ teaspoon cloves, ground
- 2 tablespoons red wine vinegar
- 1 teaspoon coriander seeds
- ½ cup water

How To:

1. Add cabbage, onion, plums, garlic, cumin, cinnamon, cloves, vinegar, coriander and water to your Slow Cooker.
2. Stir well.
3. Place lid and cook on LOW for 4 hours.
4. Divide between serving platters.
5. Enjoy!

Nutrition (Per Serving)

- Calories: 197
- Fat: 1g

- Carbohydrates: 14g
- Protein: 3g

Extreme Balsamic Chicken

Serving: 4
Prep Time: 10 minutes
Cook Time: 35 minutes
Ingredients:

- 3 boneless chicken breasts, skinless
- Sunflower seeds to taste
- ¼ cup almond flour
- 2/3 cups low-fat chicken broth
- 1 ½ teaspoons arrowroot
- ½ cup low sugar raspberry preserve
- 1 ½ tablespoons balsamic vinegar

How To:

1. Cut chicken breast into bite-sized pieces and season them with seeds.
2. Dredge the chicken pieces in flour and shake off any excess.
3. Take a non-stick skillet and place it over medium heat.
4. Add chicken to the skillet and cook for 15 minutes, making sure to turn them half-way through.
5. Remove chicken and transfer to platter.
6. Add arrowroot, broth, raspberry preserve to the skillet and stir.
7. Stir in balsamic vinegar and reduce heat to low, stir-cook for a few minutes.
8. Transfer the chicken back to the sauce and cook for 15 minutes more.
9. Serve and enjoy!

Nutrition (Per Serving)

- Calories: 546
- Fat: 35g
- Carbohydrates: 11g
- Protein: 44g

Enjoyable Spinach and Bean Medley

Serving: 4
Prep Time: 10 minutes
Cooking Time: 4 hours
Ingredients:

- 5 carrots, sliced
- 1 ½ cups great northern beans, dried
- 2 garlic cloves, minced
- 1 yellow onion, chopped
- Pepper to taste
- ½ teaspoon oregano, dried
- 5 ounces baby spinach
- 4 ½ cups low sodium veggie stock
- 2 teaspoons lemon peel, grated
- 3 tablespoon lemon juice

How To:

1. Add beans, onion, carrots, garlic, oregano and stock to your Slow Cooker.
2. Stir well.
3. Place lid and cook on HIGH for 4 hours.
4. Add spinach, lemon juice and lemon peel.
5. Stir and let it sit for 5 minutes.
6. Divide between serving platters and enjoy!

Nutrition (Per Serving)

- Calories: 219
- Fat: 8g
- Carbohydrates: 14g
- Protein: 8g

Tantalizing Cauliflower and Dill Mash

Serving: 6
Prep Time: 10 minutes
Cooking Time: 6 hours
Ingredients:

- 1 cauliflower head, florets separated
- 1/3 cup dill, chopped
- 6 garlic cloves
- 2 tablespoons olive oil
- Pinch of black pepper

How To:

1. Add cauliflower to Slow Cooker.
2. Add dill, garlic and water to cover them.
3. Place lid and cook on HIGH for 5 hours.
4. Drain the flowers.
5. Season with pepper and add oil, mash using potato masher.
6. Whisk and serve.
7. Enjoy!

Nutrition (Per Serving)

- Calories: 207
- Fat: 4g
- Carbohydrates: 14g
- Protein: 3g

Secret Asian Green Beans

Serving: 10
Prep Time: 10 minutes
Cooking Time: 2 hours
Ingredients:

- 16 cups green beans, halved
- 3 tablespoons olive oil
- ¼ cup tomato sauce, salt-free
- ½ cup coconut sugar
- ¾ teaspoon low sodium soy sauce
- Pinch of pepper

How To:

1. Add green beans, coconut sugar, pepper tomato sauce, soy sauce, oil to your Slow Cooker.
2. Stir well.
3. Place lid and cook on LOW for 3 hours.
4. Divide between serving platters and serve.
5. Enjoy!

Nutrition (Per Serving)

- Calories: 200
- Fat: 4g
- Carbohydrates: 12g
- Protein: 3g

Excellent Acorn Mix

Serving: 10
Prep Time: 10 minutes
Cooking Time: 7 hours
Ingredients:

- 2 acorn squash, peeled and cut into wedges
- 16 ounces cranberry sauce, unsweetened
- ¼ teaspoon cinnamon powder
- Pepper to taste

How To:

1. Add acorn wedges to your Slow Cooker.
2. Add cranberry sauce, cinnamon, raisins and pepper.
3. Stir.
4. Place lid and cook on LOW for 7 hours.
5. Serve and enjoy!

Nutrition (Per Serving)

- Calories: 200
- Fat: 3g
- Carbohydrates: 15g
- Protein: 2g

Crunchy Almond Chocolate Bars

Serving: 12
Prep Time: 10 minutes
Cooking Time: 2 hours 30 minutes
Ingredients:

- 1 egg white
- ¼ cup coconut oil, melted
- 1 cup coconut sugar
- ½ teaspoon vanilla extract
- 1 teaspoon baking powder
- 1 ½ cups almond meal
- ½ cup dark chocolate chips

How To:

1. Take a bowl and add sugar, oil, vanilla extract, egg white, almond flour, baking powder and mix it well.
2. Fold in chocolate chips and stir.
3. Line Slow Cooker with parchment paper.
4. Grease.
5. Add the cookie mix and press on bottom.
6. Place lid and cook on LOW for 2 hours 30 minutes.
7. Take cookie sheet out and let it cool.
8. Cut in bars and enjoy!

Nutrition (Per Serving)

- Calories: 200
- Fat: 2g
- Carbohydrates: 13g
- Protein: 6g

Lettuce and Chicken Platter

Serving: 6
Prep Time: 10 minutes
Cook Time: nil
Ingredients:

- 2 cups chicken, cooked and coarsely chopped
- ½ head ice berg lettuce, sliced and chopped
- 1 celery rib, chopped
- 1 medium apple, cut
- ½ red bell pepper, deseeded and chopped
- 6-7 green olives, pitted and halved
- 1 red onion, chopped

For dressing
- 1 tablespoon raw honey
- 2 tablespoons lemon juice
- Salt and pepper to taste

How To:

1. Cut the vegetables and transfer them to your Salad Bowl.
2. Add olives.
3. Chop the cooked chicken and transfer to your Salad bowl.
4. Prepare dressing by mixing the ingredients listed under Dressing.
5. Pour the dressing into the Salad bowl.
6. Toss and enjoy!

Nutrition (Per Serving)

- Calories: 296
- Fat: 21g
- Carbohydrates: 9g
- Protein: 18g

Greek Lemon Chicken Bowl

Serving: 6
Prep Time: 10 minutes
Cook Time: 15 minutes
Ingredients:

- 2 cups chicken, cooked and chopped
- 2 cans chicken broth, fat free
- 2 medium carrots, chopped
- ¼ teaspoon pepper
- 2 tablespoons parsley, snipped
- ¼ cup lemon juice
- 1 can cream chicken soup, fat free, low sodium
- ½ cup onion, chopped
- 1 garlic clove, minced

How To:

1. Take a pot and add all the ingredients except parsley into it.

2. Season with salt and pepper.

3. Bring the mix to a boil over medium-high heat.

4. Reduce the heat and simmer for 15 minutes.

5. Garnish with parsley.

6. Serve hot and enjoy!

Nutrition (Per Serving)

- Calories: 520
- Fat: 33g
- Carbohydrates: 31g
- Protein: 30g

Chilled Chicken, Artichoke and Zucchini Platter

Serving: 4
Prep Time: 10 minutes
Cook Time: 5 minutes
Ingredients:

- 2 medium chicken breasts, cooked and cut into 1-inch cubes
- ¼ cup extra virgin olive oil
- 2 cups artichoke hearts, drained and roughly chopped
- 3 large zucchini, diced/cut into small rounds
- 1 can (15 ounce) chickpeas
- 1 cup Kalamata olives
- ½ teaspoon Fresh ground black pepper
- ½ teaspoon Italian seasoning
- ¼ cup parmesan, grated

How To:

1. Take a large skillet and place it over medium heat, heat up olive oil.
2. Add zucchini and sauté for 5 minutes, season with salt and pepper.
3. Remove from heat and add all the listed ingredients to the skillet.
4. Stir until combined.
5. Transfer to glass container and store.
6. Serve and enjoy!

Nutrition (Per Serving)

- Calories: 457
- Fat: 22g
- Carbohydrates: 30g
- Protein: 24g

Chicken and Carrot Stew

Serving: 6
Prep Time: 15 minutes
Cook Time: 6 hours
Ingredients:

- 4 chicken breasts, boneless and cubed
- 2 cups chicken broth
- 1 cup tomatoes, chopped
- 3 cups carrots, peeled and cubed
- 1 teaspoon thyme dried
- 1 cup onion, chopped
- 2 garlic clove, minced
- Pepper to taste

How To:

1. Add all the ingredients to the Slow Cooker.

2. Stir and close the lid.

3. Cook for 6 hours.

4. Serve hot and enjoy!

Nutrition (Per Serving)

- Calories: 182
- Fat: 4g
- Carbohydrates: 10g
- Protein: 39g

Tasty Spinach Pie

Serving: 2
Prep Time: 10 minutes
Cooking Time: 4 hours
Ingredients:

- 10 ounces spinach
- 2 cups baby Bella mushrooms, chopped
- 1 red bell pepper, chopped
- 1 ½ cups low-fat cheese, shredded
- 8 whole eggs
- 1 cup coconut cream
- 2 tablespoons chives, chopped
- Pinch of pepper
- ½ cup almond flour
- ¼ teaspoon baking soda

How To:

1. Take a bowl and add eggs, coconut cream, chives, pepper and whisk well.
2. Add almond flour, baking soda, cheese, mushrooms bell pepper, spinach and toss well.
3. Grease your cooker and transfer mix to the Slow Cooker.
4. Place lid and cook on LOW for 4 hours.
5. Slice and enjoy!

Nutrition (Per Serving)

- Calories: 201
- Fat: 6g
- Carbohydrates: 8g
- Protein: 5g

Mesmerizing Carrot and Pineapple Mix

Serving: 10
Prep Time: 10 minutes
Cooking Time: 6 hours
Ingredients:

- 1 cup raisins
- 6 cups water
- 23 ounces natural applesauce
- 2 tablespoons stevia
- 2 tablespoons cinnamon powder
- 14 ounces carrots, shredded
- 8 ounces canned pineapple, crushed
- 1 tablespoon pumpkin pie spice

How To:

1. Add carrots, applesauce, raisins, stevia, cinnamon, pineapple, pumpkin pie spice to your Slow Cooker and gently stir.
2. Place lid and cook on LOW for 6 hours .
3. Serve and enjoy!

Nutrition (Per Serving)

- Calories: 179
- Fat: 5g
- Carbohydrates: 15g
- Protein: 4g

Blackberry Chicken Wings

Serving: 4
Prep Time: 35 minutes
Cook Time: 50minutes
Ingredients:

- 3 pounds chicken wings, about 20 pieces
- ½ cup blackberry chipotle jam
- Sunflower seeds and pepper to taste
- ½ cup water

How To:

1. Add water and jam to a bowl and mix well.
2. Place chicken wings in a zip bag and add two-thirds of the marinade.
3. Season with sunflower seeds and pepper.
4. Let it marinate for 30 minutes.
5. Pre-heat your oven to 400 degrees F.
6. Prepare a baking sheet and wire rack, place chicken wings in wire rack and bake for 15 minutes.
7. Brush remaining marinade and bake for 30 minutes more.
8. Enjoy!

Nutrition (Per Serving)

- Calories: 502
- Fat: 39g
- Carbohydrates: 01.8g
- Protein: 34g

Generous Lemon Dredged Broccoli

Serving: 4
Prep Time: 10 minutes
Cook Time: 15 minutes
Ingredients:

- 2 heads broccoli, separated into florets
- 2 teaspoons extra virgin olive oil
- 1 teaspoon sunflower seeds
- ½ teaspoon pepper
- 1 garlic clove, minced
- ½ teaspoon lemon juice

How To:

1. Pre-heat your oven to a temperature of 400 degrees F.

2. Take a large sized bowl and add broccoli florets with some extra virgin olive oil, pepper, sea sunflower seeds and garlic.

3. Spread the broccoli out in a single even layer on a fine baking sheet.

4. Bake in your pre-heated oven for about 15-20 minutes until the florets are soft enough to be pierced with a fork.

5. Squeeze lemon juice over them generously before serving.

6. Enjoy!

Nutrition (Per Serving)

- Calories: 49
- Fat: 2g
- Carbohydrates: 4g
- Protein: 3g

Tantalizing Almond butter Beans

Serving: 4
Prep Time: 5 minutes
Cook Time: 12 minutes
Ingredients:

- 2 garlic cloves, minced
- Red pepper flakes to taste
- Sunflower seeds to taste
- 2 tablespoons clarified butter
- 4 cups green beans, trimmed

How To:

1. Bring a pot of water to boil, with added seeds for taste.

2. Once the water starts to boil, add beans and cook for 3 minutes.

3. Take a bowl of ice water and drain beans, plunge them into the ice water.

4. Once cooled, keep them on the side.

5. Take a medium skillet and place it over medium heat, add ghee and melt.

6. Add red pepper, sunflower seeds, garlic.

7. Cook for 1 minute.

8. Add beans and toss until coated well, cook for 3 minutes.

9. Serve and enjoy!

Nutrition (Per Serving)

- Calories: 93
- Fat: 8g
- Carbohydrates: 4g
- Protein: 2g

Healthy Chicken Cream Salad

Serving: 3
Prep Time: 5 minutes
Cook Time: 50 minutes
Ingredients:

- 2 chicken breasts
- 1 ½ cups low fat cream
- 3 ounces celery
- 2 ounce green pepper, chopped
- ½ ounce green onion, chopped
- ½ cup low fat mayo
- 3 hard-boiled eggs, chopped

How To:

1. Pre-heat your oven to 350 degrees F.
2. Take a baking sheet and place chicken, cover with cream.
3. Bake for 30-40 minutes.
4. Take a bowl and mix in the chopped celery, peppers, onions.
5. Chop the baked chicken into bite-sized portions.
6. Peel and chop the hard boiled eggs.
7. Take a large salad bowl and mix in eggs, veggies and chicken.
8. Toss well and serve.
9. Enjoy!

Nutrition (Per Serving)

- Calories: 415
- Fat: 24g
- Carbohydrates: 4g
- Protein: 40g

Generously Smothered Pork Chops

Serving: 4
Prep Time: 10 minutes
Cook Time: 30 minutes
Ingredients:

- 4 pork chops, bone-in
- 2 tablespoons of olive oil
- ¼ cup vegetable broth
- ½ pound Yukon gold potatoes, peeled and chopped
- 1 large onion, sliced
- 2 garlic cloves, minced
- 2 teaspoon rubbed sage
- 1 teaspoon thyme, ground
- Pepper as needed

How To:

1. Pre-heat your oven to 350 degrees F.
2. Take a large sized skillet and place it over medium heat.
3. Add a tablespoon of oil and allow the oil to heat up.
4. Add pork chops and cook them for 4-5 minutes per side until browned.
5. Transfer chops to a baking dish.
6. Pour broth over the chops.
7. Add remaining oil to the pan and sauté potatoes, onion, garlic for 3-4 minutes.
8. Take a large bowl and add potatoes, garlic, onion, thyme, sage, pepper.
9. Transfer this mixture to the baking dish (wish pork).
10. Bake for 20-30 minutes.
11. Serve and enjoy!

Nutrition (Per Serving)

- Calorie: 261
- Fat: 10g
- Carbohydrates: 1.3g
- Protein: 2g

Crazy Lamb Salad

Serving: 4
Prep Time: 10 minutes
Cook Time: 35 minutes
Ingredients:

- 1 tablespoon olive oil
- 3 pound leg of lamb, bone removed, leg butterflied
- Salt and pepper to taste
- 1 teaspoon cumin
- Pinch of dried thyme
- 2 garlic cloves, peeled and minced

For Salad

- 4 ounces feta cheese, crumbled
- ½ cup pecans
- 2 cups spinach
- 1 ½ tablespoons lemon juice
- ¼ cup olive oil
- 1 cup fresh mint, chopped

How To:

1. Rub lamb with salt and pepper, 1 tablespoon oil, thyme, cumin, minced garlic.

2. Pre-heat your grill to medium-high and transfer lamb.

3. Cook for 40 minutes, making sure to flip it once.

4. Take a lined baking sheet and spread the pecans.

5. Toast in oven for 10 minutes at 350 degree F.

6. Transfer grilled lamb to cutting board and let it cool.

7. Slice.

8. Take a salad bowl and add spinach, 1 cup mint, feta cheese, ¼ cup olive oil, lemon juice, toasted pecans, salt, pepper and toss well.

9. Add lamb slices on top.

10. Serve and enjoy!

Nutrition (Per Serving)

- Calories: 334
- Fat: 33g
- Carbohydrates: 5g
- Protein: 7g

Hearty Roasted Cauliflower

Serving: 8
Prep Time: 5 minutes
Cook Time: 30 minutes
Ingredients:

- 1 large cauliflower head
- 2 tablespoons melted coconut oil
- 2 tablespoons fresh thyme
- 1 teaspoon Celtic sea sunflower seeds
- 1 teaspoon fresh ground pepper
- 1 head roasted garlic
- 2 tablespoons fresh thyme for garnish

How To:

1. Pre-heat your oven to 425 degrees F.
2. Rinse cauliflower and trim, core and sliced.
3. Lay cauliflower evenly on rimmed baking tray.
4. Drizzle coconut oil evenly over cauliflower, sprinkle thyme leaves .
5. Season with pinch of sunflower seeds and pepper.
6. Squeeze roasted garlic.
7. Roast cauliflower until slightly caramelized for about 30 minutes, making sure to turn once.
8. Garnish with fresh thyme leaves.
9. Enjoy!

Nutrition (Per Serving)

- Calories: 129
- Fat: 11g
- Carbohydrates: 6g
- Protein: 7g

Cool Cabbage Fried Beef

Serving: 4
Prep Time: 5 minutes
Cook Time: 15 minutes
Ingredients:

- 1 pound beef, ground and lean
- ½ pound bacon
- 1 onion
- 1 garlic cloves, minced
- ½ head cabbage
- pepper to taste

How To:

1. Take skillet and place it over medium heat.
2. Add chopped bacon, beef and onion until slightly browned.
3. Transfer to a bowl and keep it covered.
4. Add minced garlic and cabbage to the skillet and cook until slightly browned.
5. Return the ground beef mix to the skillet and simmer for 3-5 minutes over low heat.
6. Serve and enjoy!

Nutrition (Per Serving)

- Calories: 360
- Fat: 22g
- Net Carbohydrates: 5g
- Protein: 34g

Fennel and Figs Lamb

Serving: 2
Prep Time: 10 minutes
Cook Time: 40 minutes
Ingredients:

- 6 ounces lamb racks
- 1 fennel bulbs, sliced
- pepper to taste
- 1 tablespoon olive oil
- 2 figs, cut in half
- 1/8 cup apple cider vinegar
- 1/2 tablespoon swerve

How To:

1. Take a bowl and add fennel, figs, vinegar, swerve, oil and toss.
2. Transfer to baking dish.
3. Season with sunflower seeds and pepper.
4. Bake for 15 minutes at 400 degrees F.
5. Season lamb with sunflower seeds and pepper and transfer to a heated pan over medium-high heat.
6. Cook for a few minutes.
7. Add lamb to the baking dish with fennel and bake for 20 minutes.
8. Divide between plates and serve.
9. Enjoy!

Nutrition (Per Serving)

- Calories: 230
- Fat: 3g
- Carbohydrates: 5g
- Protein: 10g

Black Berry Chicken Wings

Serving: 4
Prep Time: 35 minutes
Cook Time: 50minutes
Ingredients:

- 3 pounds chicken wings, about 20 pieces
- ½ cup blackberry chipotle jam
- Pepper to taste
- ½ cup water

How To:

1. Add water and jam to a bowl and mix well.
2. Place chicken wings in a zip bag and add two-thirds of marinade.
3. Season with pepper.
4. Let it marinate for 30 minutes.
5. Pre-heat your oven to 400 degrees F.
6. Prepare a baking sheet and wire rack, place chicken wings in wire rack and bake for 15 minutes.
7. Brush remaining marinade and bake for 30 minutes more.
8. Enjoy!

Nutrition (Per Serving)

- Calories: 502
- Fat: 39g
- Carbohydrates: 01.8g
- Protein: 34g

Mushroom and Olive "Mediterranean" Steak

Serving: 2

Prep Time: 10 minutes

Cook Time: 14 minutes

Ingredients:

- 1/2 pound boneless beef sirloin steak, ¾ inch thick, cut into 4 pieces
- 1/2 large red onion, chopped
- 1/2 cup mushrooms
- 2 garlic cloves, thinly sliced
- 2 tablespoons olive oil
- 1/4 cup green olives, coarsely chopped
- 1/2 cup parsley leaves, finely cut

How To:

1. Take a large sized skillet and place it over medium-high heat.
2. Add oil and let it heat up.
3. Add beef and cook until both sides are browned, remove beef and drain fat.
4. Add the rest of the oil to the skillet and heat.
5. Add onions, garlic and cook for 2-3 minutes.
6. Stir well.
7. Add mushrooms, olives and cook until the mushrooms are thoroughly done.
8. Return the beef to the skillet and reduce heat to medium.
9. Cook for 3-4 minutes (covered).
10. Stir in parsley.
11. Serve and enjoy!

Nutrition (Per Serving)

- Calories: 386
- Fat: 30g
- Carbohydrates: 11g
- Protein: 21g

Hearty Chicken Fried Rice

Serving: 4

Prep Time: 10 minutes

Cook Time: 12 minutes

Ingredients:

- 1 teaspoon olive oil
- 4 large egg whites
- 1 onion, chopped
- 2 garlic cloves, minced
- 12 ounces skinless chicken breasts, boneless, cut into ½ inch cubes
- ½ cup carrots, chopped
- ½ cup frozen green peas
- 2 cups long grain brown rice, cooked
- 3 tablespoons soy sauce, low sodium

How To:

1. Coat skillet with oil, place it over medium-high heat.
2. Add egg whites and cook until scrambled .
3. Sauté onion, garlic and chicken breasts for 6 minutes.
4. Add carrots, peas and keep cooking for 3 minutes.
5. Stir in rice, season with soy sauce.
6. Add cooked egg whites, stir for 3 minutes.
7. Enjoy!

Nutrition (Per Serving)

- Calories: 353
- Fat: 11g
- Carbohydrates: 30g
- Protein: 23g

Chapter 3: Dinner Recipes

Decent Beef and Onion Stew

Serving: 4
Prep Time: 10 minutes
Cook Time 1-2 hours
Ingredients:

- 2 pounds lean beef, cubed
- 3 pounds shallots, peeled
- 5 garlic cloves, peeled, whole
- 3 tablespoons tomato paste
- 1 bay leaves
- ¼ cup olive oil
- 3 tablespoons lemon juice

How To:

1. Take a stew pot and place it over medium heat.
2. Add olive oil and let it heat up.
3. Add meat and brown.
4. Add remaining ingredients and cover with water.
5. Bring the whole mix to a boil.
6. Reduce heat to low and cover the pot.
7. Simmer for 1-2 hours until beef is cooked thoroughly.
8. Serve hot!

Nutrition (Per Serving)

- Calories: 136
- Fat: 3g
- Carbohydrates: 0.9g
- Protein: 24g

Clean Parsley and Chicken Breast

Serving: 2
Prep Time: 10 minutes
Cook Time: 40 minutes
Ingredients:

- 1/2 tablespoon dry parsley
- 1/2 tablespoon dry basil
- 2 chicken breast halves, boneless and skinless
- 1/4 teaspoon sunflower seeds
- 1/4 teaspoon red pepper flakes, crushed
- 1 tomato, sliced

How To:

1. Pre-heat your oven to 350 degrees F.
2. Take a 9x13 inch baking dish and grease it up with cooking spray.
3. Sprinkle 1 tablespoon of parsley, 1 teaspoon of basil and spread the mixture over your baking dish.
4. Arrange the chicken breast halves over the dish and sprinkle garlic slices on top.
5. Take a small bowl and add 1 teaspoon parsley, 1 teaspoon of basil, sunflower seeds, basil, red pepper and mix well. Pour the mixture over the chicken breast.
6. Top with tomato slices and cover, bake for 25 minutes.
7. Remove the cover and bake for 15 minutes more.
8. Serve and enjoy!

Nutrition (Per Serving)

- Calories: 150
- Fat: 4g

- Carbohydrates: 4g

- Protein: 25g

Zucchini Beef Sauté with Coriander Greens

Serving: 4
Prep Time: 10 minutes
Cook Time: 10 minutes
Ingredients:

- 10 ounces beef, sliced into 1-2 inch strips
- 1 zucchini, cut into 2-inch strips
- ¼ cup parsley, chopped
- 3 garlic cloves, minced
- 2 tablespoons tamari sauce
- 4 tablespoons avocado oil

How To:

1. Add 2 tablespoons avocado oil in a frying pan over high heat.
2. Place strips of beef and brown for a few minutes on high heat.
3. Once the meat is brown, add zucchini strips and sauté until tender.
4. Once tender, add tamari sauce, garlic, parsley and let them sit for a few minutes more.
5. Serve immediately and enjoy!

Nutrition (Per Serving)

- Calories: 500
- Fat: 40g
- Carbohydrates: 5g
- Protein: 31g

Hearty Lemon and Pepper Chicken

Serving: 4
Prep Time: 5 minutes
Cook Time: 15
Ingredients:

- 2 teaspoons olive oil
- 1 ¼ pounds skinless chicken cutlets
- 2 whole eggs
- ¼ cup panko crumbs
- 1 tablespoon lemon pepper
- Sunflower seeds and pepper to taste
- 3 cups green beans
- ¼ cup parmesan cheese
- ¼ teaspoon garlic powder

How To:

1. Pre-heat your oven to 425 degrees F.
2. Take a bowl and stir in seasoning, parmesan, lemon pepper, garlic powder, panko.
3. Whisk eggs in another bowl.
4. Coat cutlets in eggs and press into panko mix.
5. Transfer coated chicken to a parchment lined baking sheet.
6. Toss the beans in oil, pepper, add sunflower seeds, and lay them on the side of the baking sheet.
7. Bake for 15 minutes.
8. Enjoy!

Nutrition (Per Serving)

- Calorie: 299
- Fat: 10g
- Carbohydrates: 10g
- Protein: 43g

Walnuts and Asparagus Delight

Serving: 4
Prep Time: 5 minutes
Cook Time: 5 minutes
Ingredients:

- 1 ½ tablespoons olive oil
- ¾ pound asparagus, trimmed
- ¼ cup walnuts, chopped
- Sunflower seeds and pepper to taste

How To:

1. Place a skillet over medium heat add olive oil and let it heat up.
2. Add asparagus, sauté for 5 minutes until browned.
3. Season with sunflower seeds and pepper.
4. Remove heat.
5. Add walnuts and toss.
6. Serve warm!

Nutrition (Per Serving)

- Calories: 124
- Fat: 12g
- Carbohydrates: 2g
- Protein: 3g

Healthy Carrot Chips

Serving: 4
Prep Time: 10 minutes
Cook Time: 10 minutes
Ingredients:

- 3 cups carrots, sliced paper thin rounds
- 2 tablespoons olive oil
- 2 teaspoons ground cumin
- ½ teaspoon smoked paprika
- Pinch of sunflower seeds

How To:

1. Pre-heat your oven to 400 degrees F.
2. Slice carrot into paper thin shaped coins using a peeler.
3. Place slices in a bowl and toss with oil and spices.
4. Lay out the slices on a parchment paper, lined baking sheet in a single layer.
5. Sprinkle sunflower seeds.
6. Transfer to oven and bake for 8-10 minutes.
7. Remove and serve.
8. Enjoy!

Nutrition (Per Serving)

- Calories: 434
- Fat: 35g
- Carbohydrates: 31g
- Protein: 2g

Beef Soup

Serving: 4
Prep Time: 10 minutes
Cook Time: 40 minutes
Ingredients:

- 1 pound ground beef, lean
- 1 cup mixed vegetables, frozen
- 1 yellow onion, chopped
- 6 cups vegetable broth
- 1 cup low-fat cream
- Pepper to taste

How To:

1. Take a stockpot and add all the ingredients the except heavy cream, salt, and black pepper.
2. Bring to a boil.
3. Reduce heat to simmer.
4. Cook for 40 minutes.
5. Once cooked, warm the heavy cream.
6. Then add once the soup is cooked.
7. Blend the soup till smooth by using an immersion blender.
8. Season with salt and black pepper.
9. Serve and enjoy!

Nutrition (Per Serving)

- Calories: 270
- Fat: 14g
- Carbohydrates: 6g
- Protein: 29g

Amazing Grilled Chicken and Blueberry Salad

Serving: 5
Prep Time: 10 minutes
Cook Time: 25 minutes
Smart Points: 9
Ingredients:

- 5 cups mixed greens
- 1 cup blueberries
- ¼ cup slivered almonds
- 2 cups chicken breasts, cooked and cubed

For dressing

- ¼ cup olive oil
- ¼ cup apple cider vinegar
- ¼ cup blueberries
- 2 tablespoons honey
- Sunflower seeds and pepper to taste

How To:

1. Take a bowl and add greens, berries, almonds, chicken cubes and mix well.
2. Take a bowl and mix the dressing ingredients, pour the mix into a blender and blitz until smooth.
3. Add dressing on top of the chicken cubes and toss well.
4. Season more and enjoy!

Nutrition (Per Serving)

- Calories: 266
- Fat: 17g
- Carbohydrates: 18g
- Protein: 10g

Clean Chicken and Mushroom Stew

Serving: 4
Prep Time: 10 minutes
Cook Time: 35 minutes
Ingredients:

- 4 chicken breast halves, cut into bite sized pieces
- 1 pound mushrooms, sliced (5-6 cups)
- 1 bunch spring onion, chopped
- 4 tablespoons olive oil
- 1 teaspoon thyme
- Sunflower seeds and pepper as needed

How To:

1. Take a large deep frying pan and place it over medium-high heat.
2. Add oil and let it heat up.
3. Add chicken and cook for 4-5 minutes per side until slightly browned.
4. Add spring onions and mushrooms, season with sunflower seeds and pepper according to your taste.
5. Stir.
6. Cover with lid and bring the mix to a boil.
7. Reduce heat and simmer for 25 minutes.
8. Serve!

Nutrition (Per Serving)

- Calories: 247
- Fat: 12g
- Carbohydrates: 10g
- Protein: 23g

Elegant Pumpkin Chili Dish

Serving: 4
Prep Time: 10 minutes
Cook Time: 15 minutes
Ingredients:

- 3 cups yellow onion, chopped
- 8 garlic cloves, chopped
- 1 pound turkey, ground
- 2 cans (15 ounces each) fire roasted tomatoes
- 2 cups pumpkin puree
- 1 cup chicken broth
- 4 teaspoons chili spice
- 1 teaspoon ground cinnamon
- 1 teaspoon sea sunflower seeds

How To:

1. Take a large sized pot and place it over medium-high heat.
2. Add coconut oil and let the oil heat up.
3. Add onion and garlic, sauté for 5 minutes.
4. Add ground turkey and break it while cooking, cook for 5 minutes.
5. Add remaining ingredients and bring the mix to simmer.
6. Simmer for 15 minutes over low heat (lid off).
7. Pour chicken broth.
8. Serve with desired salad.
9. Enjoy!

Nutrition (Per Serving)

- Calories: 312
- Fat: 16g
- Carbohydrates: 14g
- Protein: 27g

Zucchini Zoodles with Chicken and Basil

Serving: 2
Prep Time: 10 minutes
Cook Time: 10 minutes
Ingredients:

- 2 chicken fillets, cubed
- 2 tablespoons ghee
- 1 pound tomatoes, diced
- ½ cup basil, chopped
- ¼ cup coconut almond milk
- 1 garlic clove, peeled, minced
- 1 zucchini, shredded

How To:

1. Sauté cubed chicken in ghee until no longer pink.
2. Add tomatoes and season with sunflower seeds.
3. Simmer and reduce the liquid.
4. Prepare your zucchini Zoodles by shredding zucchini in a food processor.
5. Add basil, garlic, coconut almond milk to chicken and cook for a few minutes.
6. Add half of the zucchini Zoodles to a bowl and top with creamy tomato basil chicken.
7. Enjoy!

Nutrition (Per Serving)

- Calories: 540
- Fat: 27g
- Carbohydrates: 13g
- Protein: 59g
- Fiber:
- Net Carbohydrates:

Tasty Roasted Broccoli

Serving: 4
Prep Time: 5 minutes
Cook Time: 20 minutes
Ingredients:

- 4 cups broccoli florets
- 1 tablespoon olive oil
- Sunflower seeds and pepper to taste

How To:

1. Pre-heat your oven to 400 degrees F.
2. Add broccoli in a zip bag alongside oil and shake until coated.
3. Add seasoning and shake again.
4. Spread broccoli out on baking sheet, bake for 20 minutes.
5. Let it cool and serve.
6. Enjoy!

Nutrition (Per Serving)

- Calories: 62
- Fat: 4g
- Carbohydrates: 4g
- Protein: 4g

The Almond Breaded Chicken Goodness

Serving: 3
Prep Time: 15 minutes
Cook Time: 15 minutes
Ingredients:

- 2 large chicken breasts, boneless and skinless
- 1/3 cup lemon juice
- 1 ½ cups seasoned almond meal
- 2 tablespoons coconut oil
- Lemon pepper, to taste
- Parsley for decoration

How To:

1. Slice chicken breast in half.
2. Pound out each half until ¼ inch thick.
3. Take a pan and place it over medium heat, add oil and heat it up.
4. Dip each chicken breast slice into lemon juice and let it sit for 2 minutes.
5. Turnover and the let the other side sit for 2 minutes as well.
6. Transfer to almond meal and coat both sides.
7. Add coated chicken to the oil and fry for 4 minutes per side, making sure to sprinkle lemon pepper liberally.
8. Transfer to a paper lined sheet and repeat until all chicken are fried.
9. Garnish with parsley and enjoy!

Nutrition (Per Serving)

- Calories: 325
- Fat: 24g
- Carbohydrates: 3g
- Protein: 16g

South-Western Pork Chops

Serving: 4
Prep Time: 10 minutes
Cook Time: 15 minutes
Smart Points: 3
Ingredients:

- Cooking spray as needed
- 4-ounce pork loin chop, boneless and fat rimmed
- 1/3 cup salsa
- 2 tablespoons fresh lime juice
- ¼ cup fresh cilantro, chopped

How To:

1. Take a large sized non-stick skillet and spray it with cooking spray.
2. Heat until hot over high heat.
3. Press the chops with your palm to flatten them slightly.
4. Add them to the skillet and cook on 1 minute for each side until they are nicely browned.
5. Lower the heat to medium-low.
6. Combine the salsa and lime juice.
7. Pour the mix over the chops.
8. Simmer uncovered for about 8 minutes until the chops are perfectly done.
9. If needed, sprinkle some cilantro on top.
10. Serve!

Nutrition (Per Serving)

- Calorie: 184
- Fat: 4g
- Carbohydrates: 4g
- Protein: 0.5g

Almond butter Pork Chops

Serving: 2
Prep Time: 5 minutes
Cook Time: 25 minutes
Ingredients:

- 1 tablespoon almond butter, divided
- 2 boneless pork chops
- Pepper to taste
- 1 tablespoon dried Italian seasoning, low fat and low sodium
- 1 tablespoon olive oil

How To:

1. Pre-heat your oven to 350 degrees F.
2. Pat pork chops dry with a paper towel and place them in a baking dish.
3. Season with pepper, and Italian seasoning.
4. Drizzle olive oil over pork chops.
5. Top each chop with ½ tablespoon almond butter.
6. Bake for 25 minutes.
7. Transfer pork chops on two plates and top with almond butter juice.
8. Serve and enjoy!

Nutrition (Per Serving)

- Calories: 333
- Fat: 23g
- Carbohydrates: 1g
- Protein: 31g

Chicken Salsa

Serving: 1
Prep Time: 4 minutes
Cook Time: 14 minutes
Ingredients:

- 2 chicken breasts
- 1 cup salsa
- 1 taco seasoning mix
- 1 cup plain Greek Yogurt
- ½ cup of kite ricottta/cashew cheese, cubed

How To:

1. Take a skillet and place over medium heat.
2. Add chicken breast, ½ cup of salsa and taco seasoning.
3. Mix well and cook for 12-15 minutes until the chicken is done.
4. Take the chicken out and cube them.
5. Place the cubes on toothpick and top with cheddar.
6. Place yogurt and remaining salsa in cups and use as dips.
7. Enjoy!

Nutrition (Per Serving)

- Calories: 359
- Fat: 14g
- Net Carbohydrates: 14g
- Protein: 43g

Healthy Mediterranean Lamb Chops

Serving: 4
Prep Time: 10 minutes
Cook Time: 10 minute
Ingredients:

- 4 lamb shoulder chops, 8 ounces each
- 2 tablespoons Dijon mustard
- 2 tablespoons Balsamic vinegar
- ½ cup olive oil
- 2 tablespoons shredded fresh basil

How To:

1. Pat your lamb chop dry using a kitchen towel and arrange them on a shallow glass baking dish.
2. Take a bowl and a whisk in Dijon mustard, balsamic vinegar, pepper and mix them well.
3. Whisk in the oil very slowly into the marinade until the mixture is smooth
4. Stir in basil.
5. Pour the marinade over the lamb chops and stir to coat both sides well.
6. Cover the chops and allow them to marinate for 1-4 hours (chilled).
7. Take the chops out and leave them for 30 minutes to allow the temperature to reach a normal level.
8. Pre-heat your grill to medium heat and add oil to the grate.
9. Grill the lamb chops for 5-10 minutes per side until both sides are browned.
10. Once the center reads 145 degrees F, the chops are ready, serve and enjoy!

Nutrition (Per Serving)

- Calories: 521
- Fat: 45g
- Carbohydrates: 3.5g
- Protein: 22g

Amazing Sesame Breadsticks

Serving: 5 breadsticks
Prep Time: 10 minutes
Cooking Time: 20 minutes
Ingredients:

- 1 egg white
- 2 tablespoons almond flour
- 1 teaspoon Himalayan pink sunflower seeds
- 1 tablespoon extra-virgin olive oil
- ½ teaspoon sesame seeds

How To:

1. Pre-heat your oven to 320 degrees F.
2. Line a baking sheet with parchment paper and keep it on the side.
3. Take a bowl and whisk in egg whites, add flour and half of sunflower seeds and olive oil.
4. Knead until you have a smooth dough.
5. Divide into 4 pieces and roll into breadsticks.
6. Place on prepared sheet and brush with olive oil, sprinkle sesame seeds and remaining sunflower seeds.
7. Bake for 20 minutes.
8. Serve and enjoy!

Nutrition (Per Serving)

- Total Carbs: 1.1g
- Fiber: 1g
- Protein: 1.6g
- Fat: 5g

Brown Butter Duck Breast

Serving: 3
Prep Time: 5 minutes
Cook Time: 25 minutes
Ingredients:

- 1 whole 6 ounce duck breast, skin on
- Pepper to taste
- 1 head radicchio, 4 ounces, core removed
- ¼ cup unsalted butter
- 6 fresh sage leaves, sliced

How To:

1. Pre-heat your oven to 400 degree F.
2. Pat duck breast dry with paper towel.
3. Season with pepper.
4. Place duck breast in skillet and place it over medium heat, sear for 3-4 minutes each side.
5. Turn breast over and transfer skillet to oven.
6. Roast for 10 minutes (uncovered).
7. Cut radicchio in half.
8. Remove and discard the woody white core and thinly slice the leaves.
9. Keep them on the side.
10. Remove skillet from oven.
11. Transfer duck breast, fat side up to cutting board and let it rest.
12. Re-heat your skillet over medium heat.
13. Add unsalted butter, sage and cook for 3-4 minutes.
14. Cut duck into 6 equal slices.
15. Divide radicchio between 2 plates, top with slices of duck breast and drizzle browned butter and sage.
16. Enjoy!

Nutrition (Per Serving)

- Calories: 393
- Fat: 33g
- Carbohydrates: 2g
- Protein: 22g

Generous Garlic Bread Stick

Serving: 8 breadsticks
Prep Time: 15 minutes
Cooking Time: 15 minutes
Ingredients:

- ¼ cup almond butter, softened
- 1 teaspoon garlic powder
- 2 cups almond flour
- ½ tablespoon baking powder
- 1 tablespoon Psyllium husk powder
- ¼ teaspoon sunflower seeds
- 3 tablespoons almond butter, melted
- 1 egg
- ¼ cup boiling water

How To:

1. Pre-heat your oven to 400 degrees F.
2. Line baking sheet with parchment paper and keep it on the side.
3. Beat almond butter with garlic powder and keep it on the side.
4. Add almond flour, baking powder, husk, sunflower seeds in a bowl and mix in almond butter and egg, mix well.

5. Pour boiling water in the mix and stir until you have a nice dough.
6. Divide the dough into 8 balls and roll into breadsticks.
7. Place on baking sheet and bake for 15 minutes.
8. Brush each stick with garlic almond butter and bake for 5 minutes more.
9. Serve and enjoy!

Nutrition (Per Serving)
- Total Carbs: 7g
- Fiber: 2g
- Protein: 7g
- Fat: 24g

Cauliflower Bread Stick

Serving: 5 breadsticks
Prep Time: 10 minutes
Cooking Time: 48 minutes
Ingredients:
- 1 cup cashew cheese/ kite ricotta cheese
- 1 tablespoon organic almond butter
- 1 whole egg
- ½ teaspoon Italian seasoning
- ¼ teaspoon red pepper flakes
- 1/8 teaspoon kosher sunflower seeds
- 2 cups cauliflower rice, cooked for 3 minutes in microwave
- 3 teaspoons garlic, minced
- Parmesan cheese, grated

How To:
1. Pre-heat your oven to 350 degrees F.
2. Add almond butter in a small pan and melt over low heat
3. Add red pepper flakes, garlic to the almond butter and cook for 2-3 minutes.
4. Add garlic and almond butter mix to the bowl with cooked cauliflower and add the Italian seasoning.
5. Season with sunflower seeds and mix, refrigerate for 10 minutes.
6. Add cheese and eggs to the bowl and mix.
7. Place a layer of parchment paper at the bottom of a 9 x 9 baking dish and grease with cooking spray, add egg and mozzarella cheese mix to the cauliflower mix.
8. Add mix to the pan and smooth to a thin layer with the palms of your hand.
9. Bake for 30 minutes, take out from oven and top with few shakes of parmesan and mozzarella.
10. Cook for 8 minutes more.
11. Enjoy!

Nutrition (Per Serving)
- Total Carbs: 11.5g
- Fiber: 2g
-
- Protein: 10.7g
- Fat: 20g

Bacon and Chicken Garlic Wrap

Serving: 4
Prep Time: 15 minutes
Cook Time: 10 minutes
Ingredients:

- 1 chicken fillet, cut into small cubes
- 8-9 thin slices bacon, cut to fit cubes
- 6 garlic cloves, minced

How To:

1. Pre-heat your oven to 400 degrees F.
2. Line a baking tray with aluminum foil.
3. Add minced garlic to a bowl and rub each chicken piece with it.
4. Wrap a bacon piece around each garlic chicken bite.
5. Secure with toothpick.
6. Transfer bites to baking sheet, keeping a little bit of space between them.
7. Bake for about 15-20 minutes until crispy.
8. Serve and enjoy!

Nutrition (Per Serving)

- Calories: 260
- Fat: 19g
- Carbohydrates: 5g
- Protein: 22g

Chipotle Lettuce Chicken

Serving: 6
Prep Time: 10 minutes
Cook Time: 25 minutes
Ingredients:

- 1 pound chicken breast, cut into strips
- Splash of olive oil
- 1 red onion, finely sliced
- 14 ounces tomatoes
- 1 teaspoon chipotle, chopped
- ½ teaspoon cumin
- Lettuce as needed
- Fresh coriander leaves
- Jalapeno chilies, sliced
- Fresh tomato slices for garnish
- Lime wedges

How To:

1. Take a non-stick frying pan and place it over medium heat.
2. Add oil and heat it up.
3. Add chicken and cook until brown.
4. Keep the chicken on the side.
5. Add tomatoes, sugar, chipotle, cumin to the same pan and simmer for 25 minutes until you have a nice sauce.
6. Add chicken into the sauce and cook for 5 minutes.
7. Transfer the mix to another place.
8. Use lettuce wraps to take a portion of the mixture and serve with a squeeze of lemon.
9. Enjoy!

Nutrition (Per Serving)

- Calories: 332
- Fat: 15g
- Carbohydrates: 13g
- Protein: 34g

Balsamic Chicken and Vegetables

Serving: 2
Prep Time: 15 minutes
Cook Time: 25 minutes
Ingredients:

- 4 chicken thigh, boneless and skinless
- 5 stalks of asparagus, halved
- 1 pepper, cut in chunks
- 1/2 red onion, diced
- ½ cup carrots, sliced
- 1 garlic cloves, minced
- 2-ounces mushrooms, diced
- ¼ cup balsamic vinegar
- 1 tablespoon olive oil
- ½ teaspoon stevia
- ½ tablespoon oregano
- Sunflower seeds and pepper as needed

How To:

1. Pre-heat your oven to 425 degrees F.
2. Take a bowl and add all of the vegetables and mix.
3. Add spices and oil and mix.
4. Dip the chicken pieces into spice mix and coat them well.
5. Place the veggies and chicken onto a pan in a single layer.
6. Cook for 25 minutes.
7. Serve and enjoy!

Nutrition (Per Serving)

- Calories: 401
- Fat: 17g
- Net Carbohydrates: 11g
- Protein: 48g

Cream Dredged Corn Platter

Serving: 3
Prep Time: 10 minutes
Cook Time: 4 hours
Ingredients:

- 3 cups corn
- 2 ounces cream cheese, cubed
- 2 tablespoons milk
- 2 tablespoons whipping cream
- 2 tablespoons butter, melted
- Salt and pepper as needed
- 1 tablespoon green onion, chopped

How To:

1. Add corn, cream cheese, milk, whipping cream, butter, salt and pepper to your Slow Cooker.
2. Give it a nice toss to mix everything well.
3. Place lid and cook on LOW for 4 hours.
4. Divide the mix amongst serving platters.
5. Serve and enjoy!

Nutrition (Per Serving)

- Calories: 261
- Fat: 11g
- Carbohydrates: 17g
- Protein: 6g

Exuberant Sweet Potatoes

Serving: 4
Prep Time: 5 minutes
Cook Time: 7-8 hours
Ingredients:

- 6 sweet potatoes, washed and dried

How To:

1. Loosely ball up 7-8 pieces of aluminum foil in the bottom of your Slow Cooker, covering about half of the surface area.
2. Prick each potato 6-8 times using a fork.
3. Wrap each potato with foil and seal them.
4. Place wrapped potatoes in the cooker on top of the foil bed.
5. Place lid and cook on LOW for 7-8 hours.
6. Use tongs to remove the potatoes and unwrap them.
7. Serve and enjoy!

Nutrition (Per Serving)

- Calories: 129
- Fat: 0g
- Carbohydrates: 30g
- Protein: 2g

Ethiopian Cabbage Delight

Serving: 6
Prep Time: 15 minutes
Cook Time: 6- 8 hours
Ingredients:

- ½ cup water
- 1 head green cabbage, cored and chopped
- 1 pound sweet potatoes, peeled and chopped
- 3 carrots, peeled and chopped
- 1 onion, sliced
- 1 teaspoon extra virgin olive oil
- ½ teaspoon ground turmeric
- ½ teaspoon ground cumin
- ¼ teaspoon ground ginger

How To:

1. Add water to your Slow Cooker.
2. Take a medium bowl and add cabbage, carrots, sweet potatoes, onion and mix.
3. Add olive oil, turmeric, ginger, cumin and toss until the veggies are fully coated.
4. Transfer veggie mix to your Slow Cooker.
5. Cover and cook on LOW for 6-8 hours.
6. Serve and enjoy!

Nutrition (Per Serving)

- Calories: 155
- Fat: 2g
-
- Carbohydrates: 35g
- Protein: 4g

The Vegan Lovers Refried Beans

Serving: 12
Prep Time: 5 minutes
Cook Time: 10 hours
Ingredients:

- 4 cups vegetable broth
- 4 cups water
- 3 cups dried pinto beans
- 1 onion, chopped
- 2 jalapeno peppers, minced
- 4 garlic cloves, minced
- 1 tablespoon chili powder
- 2 teaspoon ground cumin
- 1 teaspoon sweet paprika
- 1 teaspoon salt
- ½ teaspoon fresh ground black pepper

How To:
1. Add the listed ingredients to your Slow Cooker.
2. Cover and cook on HIGH for 10 hours .
3. If there's any extra liquid, ladle the liquid up and reserve it in a bowl .
4. Use an immersion blender to blend the mixture (in the Slow Cooker) until smooth.
5. Add the reserved liquid.
6. Serve hot and enjoy!

Nutrition (Per Serving)

- Calories: 91
- Fat: 0g
- Carbohydrates: 16g
- Protein: 5g

Cool Apple and Carrot Harmony

Serving: 6
Prep Time: 10 minutes
Cook Time: 10 minutes
Ingredients:

- 1 cup apple juice
- 1 pound baby carrots
- 1 tablespoon cornstarch
- 1 tablespoon mint, chopped

How To:

1. Add apple juice, carrots, cornstarch and mint to your Instant Pot.
2. Stir and lock the lid.
3. Cook on HIGH pressure for 10 minutes.
4. Perform a quick release.
5. Divide the mix amongst plates and serve.
6. Enjoy!

Nutrition (Per Serving)

- Calories: 161
- Fat: 2g
- Carbohydrates: 9g
- Protein: 8g

Mac and Chokes

Serving: 6
Prep Time: 5 minutes
Cook Time: 20 minutes
Ingredients:

- 1 tablespoon of olive oil
- 1 large sized diced onion
- 10 minced garlic cloves
- 1 can artichoke hearts
- 1 pound uncooked macaroni shells
- 12 ounce baby spinach
- 4 cups vegetable broth
- 1 teaspoon red pepper flakes
- 4 ounces vegan cheese
- ¼ cup cashew cream

How To:

1. Set the pot to Sauté mode and add oil, allow the oil to heat up and add onions.
2. Cook for 2 minutes.
3. Add garlic and stir well.
4. Add artichoke hearts and sauté for 1 minute more.
5. Add uncooked pasta and 3 cups of broth alongside 2 cups of water.
6. Mix well.
7. Lock the lid and cook on HIGH pressure for 4 minutes.
8. Quick release the pressure.
9. Open the pot and stir.
10. Add extra water, fold in spinach and cook on Sauté mode for a few minutes.
11. Add cashew cream and grated vegan cheese.
12. Add pepper flakes and mix well.
13. Enjoy!

Nutrition (Per Serving)

- Calories: 649
- Fat: 29g
- Carbohydrates: 64g
- Protein: 34g

Black Eyed Peas and Spinach Platter

Serving: 4
Prep Time: 10 minutes
Cook Time: 8 hours
Ingredients:

- 1 cup black eyed peas, soaked overnight and drained
- 2 cups low-sodium vegetable broth
- 1 can (15 ounces) tomatoes, diced with juice
- 8 ounces ham, chopped
- 1 onion, chopped
- 2 garlic cloves, minced
- 1 teaspoon dried oregano
- 1 teaspoon salt
- ½ teaspoon freshly ground black pepper
- ½ teaspoon ground mustard
- 1 bay leaf

How To:

1. Add the listed ingredients to your Slow Cooker and stir.

2. Place lid and cook on LOW for 8 hours.
3. Discard the bay leaf.
4. Serve and enjoy!

Nutrition (Per Serving)

- Calories: 209
- Fat: 6g
- Carbohydrates: 22g
- Protein: 17g

Humble Mushroom Rice

Serving: 3
Prep Time: 10 minutes
Cook Time: 3 hours
Ingredients:

- ½ cup rice
- 2 green onions chopped
- 1 garlic clove, minced
- ¼ pound baby Portobello mushrooms, sliced
- 1 cup vegetable stock

How To:
1. Add rice, onions, garlic, mushrooms, stock to your Slow Cooker.
2. Stir well and place lid.
3. Cook on LOW for 3 hours..
4. Stir and divide amongst serving platters.
5. Enjoy!

Nutrition (Per Serving)

- Calories: 200
- Fat: 6g
- Carbohydrates: 28g
- Protein: 5g

Sweet and Sour Cabbage and Apples

Serving: 4
Prep Time: 15 minutes
Cook Time: 8 hours
Ingredients:

- ¼ cup honey
- ¼ cup apple cider vinegar
- 2 tablespoons Orange Chili-Garlic Sauce
- 1 teaspoon sea salt
- 3 sweet tart apples, peeled, cored and sliced
- 2 heads green cabbage, cored and shredded
- 1 sweet red onion, thinly sliced

How To:

1. Take a small bowl and whisk in honey, orange-chili garlic sauce, vinegar.
2. Stir well.
3. Add honey mix, apples, onion and cabbage to your Slow Cooker and stir.
4. Close lid and cook on LOW for 8 hours.
5. Serve and enjoy!

Nutrition (Per Serving)
- Calories: 164
- Fat: 1g
- Carbohydrates: 41g
- Protein: 4g

Delicious Aloo Palak

Serving: 6
Prep Time: 10 minutes
Cook Time: 6-8 hours
Ingredients:

- 2 pounds red potatoes, chopped
- 1 small onion, diced
- 1 red bell pepper, seeded and diced
- ¼ cup fresh cilantro, chopped
- 1/3 cup low-sodium veggie broth
- 1 teaspoon salt
- ½ teaspoon Garam masala
- ½ teaspoon ground cumin
- ¼ teaspoon ground turmeric
- ¼ teaspoon ground coriander
- ¼ teaspoon freshly ground black pepper
- 2 pounds fresh spinach, chopped

How To:
1. Add potatoes, bell pepper, onion, cilantro, broth and seasoning to your Slow Cooker.
2. Mix well.
3. Add spinach on top.
4. Place lid and cook on LOW for 6-8 hours.
5. Stir and serve.
6. Enjoy!

Nutrition (Per Serving)
- Calories: 205
- Fat: 1g
- Carbohydrates: 44g
- Protein: 9g

Orange and Chili Garlic Sauce

Serving: 5 cups
Prep Time: 15 minutes
Cook Time: 8 hours
Ingredients:

- ½ cup apple cider vinegar
- 4 pounds red jalapeno peppers, stems, seeds and ribs removed, chopped
- 10 garlic cloves, chopped
- ½ cup tomato paste
- Juice of 1 orange zest
- ½ cup honey
- 2 tablespoons soy sauce
- 2 teaspoons salt

How To:

1. Add vinegar, garlic, peppers, tomato paste, orange juice, honey, zest, soy sauce and salt to your Slow Cooker.
2. Stir and close lid.
3. Cook on LOW for 8 hours.
4. Use as needed!

Nutrition (Per Serving)

- Calories: 33
- Fat: 1g
- Carbohydrates: 8g
- Protein: 1g

Tantalizing Mushroom Gravy

Serving: 2 cups
Prep Time: 5 minutes
Cook Time: 5-8 hours
Ingredients:

- 1 cup button mushrooms, sliced
- ¾ cup low-fat buttermilk
- 1/3 cup water
- 1 medium onion, finely diced
- 2 garlic cloves, minced
- 2 tablespoons extra virgin olive oil
- 2 tablespoons all-purpose flour
- 1 tablespoon fresh rosemary, minced
- Freshly ground black pepper

How To:

1. Add the listed ingredients to your Slow Cooker.
2. Place lid and cook on LOW for 5-8 hours.
3. Serve warm and use as needed!

Nutrition (Per Serving)

- Calories: 54
- Fat: 4g
- Carbohydrates: 4g
- Protein: 2g

Everyday Vegetable Stock

Serving: 10 cups
Prep Time: 5 minutes
Cook Time: 8-12 hours
Ingredients:

- 2 celery stalks (with leaves), quartered
- 4 ounces mushrooms, with stems
- 2 carrots, unpeeled and quartered
- 1 onion, unpeeled, quartered from pole to pole
- 1 garlic head, unpeeled, halved across middle
- 2 fresh thyme sprigs
- 10 peppercorns
- ½ teaspoon salt
- Enough water to fill 3 quarters of Slow Cooker

How To:

1. Add celery, mushrooms, onion, carrots, garlic, thyme, salt, peppercorn and water to your Slow Cooker.
2. Stir and cover .
3. Cook on LOW for 8-12 hours.
4. Strain the stock through a fine mesh cloth/metal mesh and discard solids.
5. Use as needed.

Nutrition (Per Serving)

- Calories: 38
- Fat: 5g
- Carbohydrates: 1g
- Protein: 0g

Grilled Chicken with Lemon and Fennel

Serving: 4
Prep Time: 5 minutes
Cook Time: 25 minutes
Ingredients:

- 2 cups chicken fillets , cut and skewed
- 1 large fennel bulb
- 2 garlic cloves
- 1 jar green olives
- 1 lemon

How To:

1. Pre-heat your grill to medium-high.
2. Crush garlic cloves.
3. Take a bowl and add olive oil and season with sunflower seeds and pepper.
4. Coat chicken skewers with the marinade.
5. Transfer them under the grill and grill for 20 minutes, making sure to turn them halfway through until golden.
6. Zest half of the lemon and cut the other half into quarters.
7. Cut the fennel bulb into similarly sized segments.
8. Brush olive oil all over the garlic clove segments and cook for 3-5 minutes.
9. Chop them and add them to the bowl with the marinade.
10. Add lemon zest and olives.
11. Once the meat is ready, serve with the vegetable mix.
12. Enjoy!

Nutrition (Per Serving)

- Calories: 649
- Fat: 16g
- Carbohydrates: 33g
- Protein: 18g

Caramelized Pork Chops and Onion

Serving: 4
Prep Time: 5 minutes
Cook Time: 40 minutes
Ingredients:

- 4 ounces green Chili, chopped
- 2 tablespoons of chili powder
- ½ teaspoon of dried oregano
- ½ teaspoon of cumin, ground
- 2 garlic cloves, minced
- 4-pound chuck roast

How To:

1. Rub the chops with a seasoning of 1 teaspoon of pepper and 2 teaspoons of sunflower seeds.
2. Take a skillet and place it over medium heat, add oil and allow the oil to heat up
3. Brown the seasoned chop both sides.
4. Add water and onion to the skillet and cover, lower the heat to low and simmer for 20 minutes.
5. Turn the chops over and season with more sunflower seeds and pepper.
6. Cover and cook until the water fully evaporates and the beer shows a slightly brown texture.
7. Remove the chops and serve with a topping of the caramelized onion.
8. Serve and enjoy!

Nutrition (Per Serving)

- Calorie: 47
- Fat: 4g
- Carbohydrates: 4g
- Protein: 0.5g

Hearty Pork Belly Casserole

Serving: 4
Prep Time: 5 minutes
Cook Time: 25 minutes
Ingredients:

- 8 pork belly slices, cut into small pieces
- 3 large onions, chopped
- 4 tablespoons lemon
- Juice of 1 lemon
- Seasoning as you needed

How To:

1. Take a large pressure cooker and place it over medium heat.
2. Add onions and sweat them for 5 minutes.
3. Add pork belly slices and cook until the meat browns and onions become golden.
4. Cover with water and add honey, lemon zest, sunflower seeds, pepper, and close the pressure seal.
5. Pressure cook for 40 minutes.
6. Serve and enjoy with a garnish of fresh chopped parsley if you prefer.

Nutrition (Per Serving)

- Calories: 753
- Fat: 41g
- Carbohydrates: 68g
- Protein: 30g

Apple Pie Crackers

Serving: 100 crackers
Prep Time: 10 minutes
Cooking Time: 120 minutes
Ingredients:

- 2 tablespoons + 2 teaspoons avocado oil
- 1 medium Granny Smith apple, roughly chopped
- ¼ cup Erythritol
- 1/4 cup sunflower seeds, ground
- 1 ¾ cups roughly ground flax seeds
- 1/8 teaspoon Ground cloves
- 1/8 teaspoon ground cardamom
- 3 tablespoons nutmeg
- ¼ teaspoon ground ginger

How To:

1. Pre-heat your oven to 225 degrees F.
2. Line two baking sheets with parchment paper and keep them on the side.
3. Add oil, apple, Erythritol to a bowl and mix.
4. Transfer to food processor and add remaining ingredients, process until combined.
5. Transfer batter to baking sheets, spread evenly and cut into crackers.
6. Bake for 1 hour, flip and bake for another hour.
7. Let them cool and serve.
8. Enjoy!

Nutrition (Per Serving)

- Total Carbs: 0.9g (%)
- Fiber: 0.5g
- Protein: 0.4g (%)
- Fat: 2.1g (%)

Paprika Lamb Chops

Serving: 4
Prep Time: 10 minutes
Cook Time: 15 minutes
Ingredients:

- 1 lamb rack, cut into chops
- pepper to taste
- 1 tablespoon paprika
- 1/2 cup cumin powder
- 1/2 teaspoon chili powder

How To:

1. Take a bowl and add paprika, cumin, chili, pepper, and stir.
2. Add lamb chops and rub the mixture.
3. Heat grill over medium-temperature and add lamb chops, cook for 5 minutes.
4. Flip and cook for 5 minutes more, flip again.
5. Cook for 2 minutes, flip and cook for 2 minutes more.
6. Serve and enjoy!

Nutrition (Per Serving)

- Calories: 200
- Fat: 5g
- Carbohydrates: 4g
- Protein: 8g

Chapter 4: Dessert Recipes

Hearty Chia and Blackberry Pudding

Serving: 2
Prep Time: 45 minutes
Cook Time: Nil
Ingredients:

- ¼ cup chia seeds
- ½ cup blackberries, fresh
- 1 teaspoon liquid sweetener
- 1 cup coconut almond milk, full fat and unsweetened
- 1 teaspoon vanilla extract

How To:

1. Take the vanilla, liquid sweetener and coconut almond milk and add to blender.
2. Process until thick.
3. Add in blackberries and process until smooth.
4. Divide the mixture between cups and chill for 30 minutes.
5. Serve and enjoy!

Nutrition (Per Serving)

- Calories: 437
- Fat: 38g
- Carbohydrates: 8g
- Protein: 8g

Special Cocoa Brownie Bombs

Serving: 12
Prep Time: 15 minutes
Cooking Time: 25 minutes
Freeze Time: None
Ingredients:

- 2 tablespoons grass-fed almond butter
- 1 whole egg
- 2 teaspoons vanilla extract
- ¼ teaspoon baking powder
- 1/3 cup heavy cream
- 3/4 cup almond butter
- ¼ cocoa powder
- A pinch of sunflower seeds

How To:

1. Break the eggs and whisk until smooth.
2. Add in all the wet ingredients and mix well.
3. Make the batter by mixing all the dry ingredients and sifting them into the wet ingredients.
4. Pour into a greased baking pan.
5. Bake for 25 minutes at 350 degrees F or until a toothpick inserted in the middle comes out clean.
6. Let it cool, slice and serve.

Nutrition (Per Serving)

- Total Carbs: 1g
- Fiber: 0g
- Protein: 1g
- Fat: 20g

Gentle Blackberry Crumble

Serving: 4
Prep Time: 10 minutes
Cook Time: 45 minutes
Smart Points: 4
Ingredients:

- ½ cup coconut flour
- ½ cup banana, peeled and mashed
- 6 tablespoons water
- 3 cups fresh blackberries
- ½ cup arrowroot flour
- 1 ½ teaspoons baking soda
- 4 tablespoons almond butter, melted
- 1 tablespoon fresh lemon juice

How To:

1. Pre-heat your oven to 300 degrees F.
2. Take a baking dish and grease it lightly.
3. Take a bowl and mix all of the ingredients except the blackberries, mix well.
4. Place blackberries in the bottom of your baking dish and top with flour.
5. Bake for 40 minutes.
6. Serve and enjoy!

Nutrition (Per Serving)

- Calories: 12
- Fat: 7g
- Carbohydrates: 10g
- Protein: 4g

Mini Minty Happiness

Serving: 12
Prep Time: 45 minutes
Cooking Time: None
Freeze Time: 2 hours
Ingredients:

- 2 teaspoons vanilla extract
- 1 ½ cups coconut oil
- 1 ¼ cups sunflower seed almond butter
- ½ cup dried parsley
- 1 teaspoon peppermint extract
- A pinch of sunflower seeds
- 1 cup dark chocolate chips
- Stevia to taste

How To:

1. Melt together coconut oil and dark chocolate chips over a double boiler.
2. Take a food processor, add all the ingredients into it and pulse until smooth.
3. Pour into round molds.
4. Let it freeze.

Nutrition (Per Serving)

- Total Carbs: 7g
- Fiber: 1g
- Protein: 3g
- Fat: 25g

Astonishing Maple Pecan Bacon Slices

Serving: 12
Prep Time: 10 minutes
Cooking Time: 25 minutes
Freeze Time: None
Ingredients:

- 1 tablespoon sugar-free maple syrup
- 12 bacon slices

For the coating:

- 4 tablespoons dark cocoa powder
- ¼ cup pecans, chopped

- Granulated Stevia to taste
- 15-20 drops Stevia

- 15-20 drops Stevia

How To:

1. Take a baking tray and lay the bacon slices on it.
2. Rub with maple syrup and Stevia, flip the slices and do the same with the other side.
3. Bake for 10-15 minutes at 227 degrees F.
4. After they've baked, drain the bacon grease.
5. To form a batter, mix the bacon grease, Stevia and cocoa powder.
6. Dip the bacon slices into the batter and roll in the chopped pecans.
7. Allow to air dry until the chocolate hardens.

Nutrition (Per Serving)

- Total Carbs: 1g
- Fiber: 0g

- Protein: 10g
- Fat: 11g

Generous Maple and Pecan Bites

Serving: 12
Prep Time: 10 minutes
Cooking Time: 25 minutes
Freeze Time: None
Ingredients:

- 1 cup almond meal
- ½ cup coconut oil
- ½ cup flaxseed meal
- ½ cup sugar-free chocolate chips

- 2 cups pecans, chopped
- ½ cup sugar-free maple syrup
- 20-25 drops Stevia

How To:

1. Take a baking dish and spread the pecans.
2. Bake at 350 degrees F until aromatic.
3. This will usually take from 6 to 8 minutes.
4. Meanwhile, sift together all the dry ingredients.
5. Add the roasted pecans to the mix and mix them properly.
6. Add the coconut oil and maple syrup.
7. Stir to make a thick, sticky mixture.
8. Take a bread pan lined with parchment paper, and pour the mixture into it.
9. Bake for about 18 minutes.
10. Slice and serve.

Nutrition (Per Serving)

- Total Carbs: 6g
- Fiber: 0g

- Protein: 5g
- Fat: 30g

Carrot Ball Delight

Serving: 4
Prep Time: 10 minutes
Cook Time: Nil
Smart Points: 2
Ingredients:

- 6 Medjool dates pitted
- 1 carrot, finely grated
- ¼ cup raw walnuts
- ¼ cup unsweetened coconut, shredded
- 1 teaspoon nutmeg
- 1/8 teaspoon sunflower seeds

How To:

1. Take a food processor and add dates, ¼ cup of grated carrots, sunflower seeds coconut, nutmeg.
2. Mix well and puree the mixture.
3. Add the walnuts and remaining ¼ cup of carrots.
4. Pulse the mixture until you have a chunky texture.
5. Form balls using your hand and roll them up in coconut.
6. Top with carrots and chill.
7. Enjoy!

Nutrition (Per Serving)

- Calories: 326
- Fat: 16g
- Carbohydrates: 42g
- Protein: 3g

Awesome Brownie Muffins

Serving: 5
Prep Time: 10 minutes
Cooking Time: 35 minutes
Ingredients:

- 1 cup golden flaxseed meal
- ¼ cup cocoa powder
- 1 tablespoon cinnamon
- ½ tablespoon baking powder
- ½ teaspoon sunflower seeds
- 1 whole large egg
- 2 tablespoons coconut oil
- ¼ cup sugar-free caramel syrup
- ½ cup pumpkin puree
- 1 teaspoon vanilla extract
- 1 teaspoon apple cider vinegar
- ¼ cup almonds, slivered

How To:

1. Pre-heat your oven to 350 degrees F.

2. Take a mixing bowl and add all of the listed ingredients and mix everything well.

3. Take your desired number of muffin tins and line them with paper liners.

4. Scoop the batter into the muffin tins, filling them to about 1/4 of the liner.

5. Sprinkle a bit of almond on top.

6. Place them in your oven and bake for 15 minutes.

7. Serve warm.

Nutrition (Per Serving)

- Total Carbs: 16
- Fiber: 2g
- Protein: 3g
- Fat: 31g

Spice Friendly Muffins

Serving: 12
Prep Time: 5 minutes
Cooking Time: 45minute
Ingredients:

- ½ cup raw hemp hearts
- ½ cup flaxseeds
- ¼ cup chia seeds
- 2 tablespoons Psyllium husk powder
- 1 tablespoon cinnamon
- Stevia taste
- ½ teaspoon baking powder
- ½ teaspoon sunflower seeds
- 1 cup of water

How To:

1. Pre-heat your oven to 350 degrees F.

2. Line muffin tray with liners.

3. Take a large sized mixing bowl and add peanut almond butter, pumpkin, sweetener, coconut almond milk, flaxseed and mix well.

4. Keep stirring until the mixture has been thoroughly combined.

5. Take another bowl and add baking powder, spices and coconut flour.

6. Mix well.

7. Add the dry ingredients into the wet bowl and stir until the coconut flour has mixed well.

8. Allow it to sit for a while until the coconut flour has absorbed all of the moisture.

9. Divide the mixture amongst your muffin tins and bake for 45 minutes.

10. Enjoy!

Nutrition (Per Serving)

- Total Carbs: 7g
- Fiber: 3g
- Protein: 6g
- Fat: 15g

Simple Gingerbread Muffins

Serving: 12
Prep Time: 5 minutes
Cooking Time: 30 minutes
Ingredients:

- 1 tablespoon ground flaxseed
- 6 tablespoons coconut almond milk
- 1 tablespoon apple cider vinegar
- ½ cup peanut almond butter
- 2 tablespoons gingerbread spice blend
- 1 teaspoon baking powder
- 1 teaspoon vanilla extract
- 2 tablespoons Swerve

How To:

1. Pre-heat your oven to 350 degrees F.
2. Take a bowl and add flaxseeds, sweetener, sunflower seeds, vanilla, spices and your non-dairy almond milk.
3. Keep it on the side for a while.
4. Add peanut almond butter, baking powder and keep mixing until combined well.
5. Stir in peanut almond butter and baking powder.
6. Mix well.
7. Spoon the mixture into muffin liners.
8. Bake for 30 minutes.
9. Allow them to cool and enjoy!

Nutrition (Per Serving)

- Total Carbs: 13g
- Fiber: 4g
- Protein: 11g
- Fat: 23g

Fantastic Cauliflower Bagels

Serving: 12
Prep Time: 10 minutes
Cooking Time: 30 minutes
Ingredients:

- 1 large cauliflower, divided into florets and roughly chopped
- ¼ cup nutritional yeast
- ¼ cup almond flour
- ½ teaspoon garlic powder
- 1 ½ teaspoon fine sea sunflower seeds
- 1 whole egg
- 1 tablespoon sesame seeds

How To:

1. Pre-heat your oven to 400 degrees F.
2. Line a baking sheet with parchment paper, keep it on the side.
3. Blend cauliflower in the food processor and transfer to a bowl.
4. Add nutritional yeast, almond flour, garlic powder and sunflower seeds to a bowl, mix.
5. Take another bowl and whisk in eggs, add to cauliflower mix.
6. Give the dough a stir.
7. Incorporate the mix into the egg mix.
8. Make balls from dough, making a hole using your thumb into each ball.
9. Arrange them on your prepped sheet, flattening them into bagel shapes.
10. Sprinkle sesame seeds and bake for 30 minutes.
11. Remove oven and let them cool, enjoy!

Nutrition (Per Serving)

- Total Carbs: 1.5g
- Fiber: 1g
- Protein: 2g
- Fat: 5.8g

Nutmeg Nougats

Serving: 12
Prep Time: 10 minutes
Cooking Time: 5 minutes
Freeze Time: 30 minutes
Ingredients:

- 1 cup coconut, shredded
- 1 cup low-fat cream
- 1 cup cashew almond butter
- ½ teaspoon ground nutmeg

How To:

1. Melt the cashew almond butter over a double boiler.
2. Stir in nutmeg and dairy cream.
3. Remove from the heat.
4. Allow to cool down a little.
5. Keep in the refrigerator for at least 30 minutes.
6. Take out from the fridge and make small balls.
7. Coat with shredded coconut.
8. Let it cool for 2 hours and then serve.

Nutrition (Per Serving)

- Total Carbs: 13g
- Fiber: 8g
- Protein: 3g
- Fat: 34g

Limey Savory Pie

Serving: 12
Prep Time: 5 minutes
Cooking Time: 5 minutes
Freeze Time: 2 hours
Ingredients:

- 1 tablespoon ground cinnamon
- 3 tablespoons almond butter
- 1 cup almond flour

For the filling:

- 3 tablespoons grass-fed almond butter
- 4 ounces full-fat cream cheese
- ¼ cup coconut oil
- 2 limes
- A handful of baby spinach
- Stevia to taste

How To:

1. Mix cinnamon and almond butter to form a crumble mixture.
2. Press this mixture into the bottom of 12 muffin cups.
3. Bake for 7 minutes at 350 degrees F.
4. Juice the lime and grate for zest while the crust is baking.
5. Take a food processor and add all the filling ingredients.
6. Blend until smooth.
7. Let it cool naturally.
8. Pour the mixture in the center.
9. Freeze until set and serve.

Nutrition (Per Serving)

- Total Carbs: 2g
- Fiber: 1g
- Protein: 3g
- Fat: 1g

Supreme Raspberry Chocolate Bombs

Serving: 6
Prep Time: 10 minutes
Cooking Time: /
Freeze Time: 1 hour
Ingredients:

- ½ cacao almond butter
- ½ coconut manna
- 4 tablespoons powdered coconut almond milk
- 3 tablespoons granulated stevia
- ¼ cup dried and crushed raspberries, frozen

How To:

1. Prepare your double boiler to medium heat and melt the cacao almond butter and coconut manna.
2. Stir in vanilla extract.
3. Take another dish and add coconut powder and sugar substitute.
4. Stir the coconut mix into the cacao almond butter, 1 tablespoon at a time, making sure to keep mixing after each addition.
5. Add the crushed dried raspberries.
6. Mix well and portion it out into muffin tins.
7. Chill for 60 minutes and enjoy!

Nutrition (Per Serving)

- Total Carbs: 7g
- Fiber: 1g
- Protein: 11g
- Fat: 21g

The Perfect Orange Ponzu

Serving: 8
Prep Time: 30 minutes
Cook Time: 5 minutes
Ingredients:

- ¼ cup coconut aminos
- ½ cup rice vinegar
- 2 tablespoons dry fish flakes
- 1 (1 inch) square kombu (kelp)
- 1 orange, quartered

How To:

1. Take a saucepan and place it over medium heat.
2. Add coconut aminos, rice vinegar, fish flakes, kombu, orange quarters and let the mixture sit for 30 minutes.
3. Bring the mix to a boil and immediately remove from the heat.
4. Let it cool and strain through a cheesecloth.
5. Serve and enjoy!

Nutrition (Per Serving)

- Calories: 15
- Fat: 0g
- Carbohydrates: 4g
- Protein: 0.8g

Hearty Cashew and Almond butter

Serving: 1 and ½ cups
Prep Time: 5 minutes
Cook Time: Nil
Ingredients:

- 1 cup almonds, blanched
- 1/3 cup cashew nuts
- 2 tablespoons coconut oil
- Sunflower seeds as needed
- ½ teaspoon cinnamon

How To:

1. Pre-heat your oven to 350 degrees F.
2. Bake almonds and cashews for 12 minutes.
3. Let them cool.
4. Transfer to food processor and add remaining ingredients.
5. Add oil and keep blending until smooth.
6. Serve and enjoy!

Nutrition (Per Serving)

- Calories: 205
- Fat: 19g
- Carbohydrates: g
- Protein: 2.8g

The Refreshing Nutter

Serving: 1
Prep Time: 10 minutes
Ingredients:

- 1 tablespoon chia seeds
- 2 cups water
- 1 ounces Macadamia Nuts
- 1-2 packets Stevia, optional
- 1 ounce hazelnut

How To:

1. Add all the listed ingredients to a blender.
2. Blend on high until smooth and creamy.
3. Enjoy your smoothie.

Nutrition (Per Serving)

- Calories: 452
- Fat: 43g
- Carbohydrates: 15g
- Protein: 9g

Elegant Cranberry Muffins

Serving: 24 muffins
Prep Time: 10 minutes
Cooking Time: 20 minutes
Ingredients:

- 2 cups almond flour
- 2 teaspoons baking soda
- ¼ cup avocado oil
- 1 whole egg
- ¾ cup almond milk
- ½ cup Erythritol
- ½ cup apple sauce
- Zest of 1 orange
- 2 teaspoons ground cinnamon
- 2 cup fresh cranberries

How To:

1. Pre-heat your oven to 350 degrees F.
2. Line muffin tin with paper muffin cups and keep them on the side.
3. Add flour, baking soda and keep it on the side.
4. Take another bowl and whisk in remaining ingredients and add flour, mix well.
5. Pour batter into prepared muffin tin and bake for 20 minutes.
6. Once done, let it cool for 10 minutes.
7. Serve and enjoy!

Nutrition (Per Serving)

- Total Carbs: 7g
- Fiber: 2g
- Protein: 2.3g
- Fat: 7g

Apple and Almond Muffins

Serving: 6 muffins
Prep Time: 10 minutes
Cooking Time: 20 minutes
Ingredients:

- 6 ounces ground almonds
- 1 teaspoon cinnamon
- ½ teaspoon baking powder
- 1 pinch sunflower seeds
- 1 whole egg
- 1 teaspoon apple cider vinegar
- 2 tablespoons Erythritol
- 1/3 cup apple sauce

How To:

1. Pre-heat your oven to 350 degrees F.
2. Line muffin tin with paper muffin cups, keep them on the side.
3. Mix in almonds, cinnamon, baking powder, sunflower seeds and keep it on the side.
4. Take another bowl and beat in eggs, apple cider vinegar, apple sauce, Erythritol.
5. Add the mix to dry ingredients and mix well until you have a smooth batter.
6. Pour batter into tin and bake for 20 minutes.
7. Once done, let them cool.
8. Serve and enjoy!

Nutrition (Per Serving)

- Total Carbs: 10
- Fiber: 4g
- Protein: 13g
- Fat: 17g

- ## **Stylish Chocolate Parfait**

Serving: 4
Prep Time: 2 hours
Cook Time: nil
Ingredients:

- 2 tablespoons cocoa powder
- 1 cup almond milk
- 1 tablespoon chia seeds
- Pinch of sunflower seeds
- ½ teaspoon vanilla extract

How To:

1. Take a bowl and add cocoa powder, almond milk, chia seeds, vanilla extract and stir.
2. Transfer to dessert glass and place in your fridge for 2 hours.
3. Serve and enjoy!

Nutrition (Per Serving)

- Calories: 130
- Fat: 5g
- Carbohydrates: 7g
- Protein: 16g

Supreme Matcha Bomb

Serving: 10
Prep Time: 100 minutes
Cook Time: Nil
Ingredients:

- 3/4 cup hemp seeds
- ½ cup coconut oil
- 2 tablespoons coconut almond butter
- 1 teaspoon Matcha powder
- 2 tablespoons vanilla bean extract
- ½ teaspoon mint extract
- Liquid stevia

How To:

1. Take your blender/food processor and add hemp seeds, coconut oil, Matcha, vanilla extract and stevia.
2. Blend until you have a nice batter and divide into silicon molds.
3. Melt coconut almond butter and drizzle on top.
4. Let the cups chill and enjoy!

Nutrition (Per Serving)

- Calories: 200
- Fat: 20g
- Carbohydrates: 3g
- Protein: 5g

Mesmerizing Avocado and Chocolate Pudding

Serving: 2
Prep Time: 30 minutes
Cook Time: Nil
Ingredients:

- 1 avocado, chunked
- 1 tablespoon natural sweetener such as stevia
- 2 ounces cream cheese, at room temp
- ¼ teaspoon vanilla extract
- 4 tablespoons cocoa powder, unsweetened

How To:

1. Blend listed ingredients in blender until smooth.
2. Divide the mix between dessert bowls, chill for 30 minutes.
3. Serve and enjoy!

Nutrition (Per Serving)

- Calories: 281
- Fat: 27g
- Carbohydrates: 12g
- Protein: 8g

Hearty Pineapple Pudding

Serving: 4
Prep Time: 10 minutes
Cooking Time: 5 hours
Ingredients:

- 1 teaspoon baking powder
- 1 cup coconut flour
- 3 tablespoons stevia
- 3 tablespoons avocado oil
- ½ cup coconut milk
- ½ cup pecans, chopped
- ½ cup pineapple, chopped
- ½ cup lemon zest, grated
- 1 cup pineapple juice, natural

How To:

1. Grease Slow Cooker with oil.
2. Take a bowl and mix in flour, stevia, baking powder, oil, milk, pecans, pineapple, lemon zest, pineapple juice and stir well.
3. Pour the mix into the Slow Cooker.
4. Place lid and cook on LOW for 5 hours.
5. Divide between bowls and serve.
6. Enjoy!

Nutrition (Per Serving)

- Calories: 188
- Fat: 3g
- Carbohydrates: 14g
- Protein: 5g

Healthy Berry Cobbler

Serving: 8
Prep Time: 10 minutes
Cooking Time: 2 hours 30 minutes
Ingredients:

- 1 ¼ cups almond flour
- 1 cup coconut sugar
- 1 teaspoon baking powder
- ½ teaspoon cinnamon powder
- 1 whole egg
- ¼ cup low-fat milk
- 2 tablespoons olive oil
- 2 cups raspberries
- 2 cups blueberries

How To:

1. Take a bowl and add almond flour, coconut sugar, baking powder and cinnamon.
2. Stir well .
3. Take another bowl and add egg, milk, oil, raspberries, blueberries and stir.
4. Combine both of the mixtures.
5. Grease your Slow Cooker.
6. Pour the combined mixture into your Slow Cooker and cook on HIGH for 2 hours 30 minutes.
7. Divide between serving bowls and enjoy!

Nutrition (Per Serving)

- Calories: 250
- Fat: 4g
- Carbohydrates: 30g
- Protein: 3g

Tasty Poached Apples

Serving: 8
Prep Time: 10 minutes
Cooking Time: 2 hours 30 minutes
Ingredients:

- 6 apples, cored, peeled and sliced
- 1 cup apple juice, natural
- 1 cup coconut sugar
- 1 tablespoon cinnamon powder

How To:

1. Grease Slow Cooker with cooking spray.
2. Add apples, sugar, juice, cinnamon to your Slow Cooker.
3. Stir gently.
4. Place lid and cook on HIGH for 4 hours.
5. Serve cold and enjoy!

Nutrition (Per Serving)

- Calories: 180
- Fat: 5g
- Carbohydrates: 8g
- Protein: 4g

Home Made Trail Mix For The Trip

Serving: 4
Prep Time: 10 minutes
Cook Time: 55 minutes
Ingredients:

- ¼ cup raw cashews
- ¼ cup almonds
- ¼ cup walnuts
- 1 teaspoon cinnamon
- 2 tablespoons melted coconut oil
- Sunflower seeds as needed

How To:

1. Line baking sheet with parchment paper.
2. Pre-heat your oven to 275 degrees F.
3. Melt coconut oil and keep it on the side.
4. Combine nuts to large mixing bowl and add cinnamon and melted coconut oil.
5. Stir.
6. Sprinkle sunflower seeds.
7. Place in oven and brown for 6 minutes.
8. Enjoy!

Nutrition (Per Serving)

- Calories: 363
- Fat: 22g
- Carbohydrates: 41g
- Protein: 7g

Heart Warming Cinnamon Rice Pudding

Serving: 4
Prep Time: 10 minutes
Cooking Time: 5 hours
Ingredients:

- 6 ½ cups water
- 1 cup coconut sugar
- 2 cups white rice
- 2 cinnamon sticks
- ½ cup coconut, shredded

How To:

1. Add water, rice, sugar, cinnamon and coconut to your Slow Cooker.
2. Gently stir.
3. Place lid and cook on HIGH for 5 hours.
4. Discard cinnamon.
5. Divide pudding between dessert dishes and enjoy!

Nutrition (Per Serving)

- Calories: 173
- Fat: 4g
- Carbohydrates: 9g
- Protein: 4g

Pure Avocado Pudding

Serving: 4
Prep Time: 3 hours
Cook Time: nil
Ingredients:

- 1 cup almond milk
- 2 avocados, peeled and pitted
- ¾ cup cocoa powder
- 1 teaspoon vanilla extract
- 2 tablespoons stevia
- ¼ teaspoon cinnamon
- Walnuts, chopped for serving

How To:

1. Add avocados to a blender and pulse well.

2. Add cocoa powder, almond milk, stevia, vanilla bean extract and pulse the mixture well.

3. Pour into serving bowls and top with walnuts.

4. Chill for 2-3 hours and serve!

Nutrition (Per Serving)

- Calories: 221
- Fat: 8g
- Carbohydrates: 7g
- Protein: 3g

Sweet Almond and Coconut Fat Bombs

Serving: 6
Prep Time: 10 minutes
Cooking Time: /
Freeze Time: 20 minutes
Ingredients:

- ¼ cup melted coconut oil
- 9 ½ tablespoons almond butter
- 90 drops liquid stevia
- 3 tablespoons cocoa
- 9 tablespoons melted almond butter, sunflower seeds

How To:

1. Take a bowl and add all of the listed ingredients.

2. Mix them well.

3. Pour 2 tablespoons of the mixture into as many muffin molds as you like.

4. Chill for 20 minutes and pop them out.

5. Serve and enjoy!

Nutrition (Per Serving)

- Total Carbs: 2g
- Fiber: 0g
- Protein: 2.53g
- Fat: 14g

Spicy Popper Mug Cake

Serving: 2
Prep Time: 5 minutes
Cook Time: 5 minutes

Ingredients:

- 2 tablespoons almond flour
- 1 tablespoon flaxseed meal
- 1 tablespoon almond butter
- 1 tablespoon cream cheese
- 1 large egg
- 1 bacon, cooked and sliced
- ½ jalapeno pepper
- ½ teaspoon baking powder
- ¼ teaspoon sunflower seeds

How To:

1. Take a frying pan and place it over medium heat.
2. Add slice of bacon and cook until it has a crispy texture.
3. Take a microwave proof container and mix all of the listed ingredients (including cooked bacon), clean the sides.
4. Microwave for 75 seconds, making to put your microwave to high power.
5. Take out the cup and tap it against a surface to take the cake out.
6. Garnish with a bit of jalapeno and serve!

Nutrition (Per Serving)

- Calories: 429
- Fat: 38g
- Carbohydrates: 6g
- Protein: 16g

The Most Elegant Parsley Soufflé Ever

Serving: 5
Prep Time: 5 minutes
Cook Time: 6 minutes
Ingredients:

- 2 whole eggs
- 1 fresh red chili pepper, chopped
- 2 tablespoons coconut cream
- 1 tablespoon fresh parsley, chopped
- Sunflower seeds to taste

How To:

1. Pre-heat your oven to 390 degrees F.
2. Almond butter 2 soufflé dishes.
3. Add the ingredients to a blender and mix well.
4. Divide batter into soufflé dishes and bake for 6 minutes.
5. Serve and enjoy!

Nutrition (Per Serving)

- Calories: 108
- Fat: 9g
- Carbohydrates: 9g
- Protein: 6g

Fennel and Almond Bites

Serving: 12
Prep Time: 10 minutes
Cooking Time: None
Freeze Time: 3 hours
Ingredients:

- 1 teaspoon vanilla extract
- ¼ cup almond milk
- ¼ cup cocoa powder
- ½ cup almond oil
- A pinch of sunflower seeds
- 1 teaspoon fennel seeds

How To:

1. Take a bowl and mix the almond oil and almond milk.
2. Beat until smooth and glossy using electric beater.
3. Mix in the rest of the ingredients.
4. Take a piping bag and pour into a parchment paper lined baking sheet.
5. Freeze for 3 hours and store in the fridge.

Nutrition (Per Serving)

- Total Carbs: 1g
- Fiber: 1g
- Protein: 1g
- Fat: 20g

Feisty Coconut Fudge

Serving: 12
Prep Time: 20 minutes
Cooking Time: None
Freeze Time: 2 hours
Ingredients:

- ¼ cup coconut, shredded
- 2 cups coconut oil
- ½ cup coconut cream
- ¼ cup almonds, chopped
- 1 teaspoon almond extract
- A pinch of sunflower seeds
- Stevia to taste

How To:

1. Take a large bowl and pour coconut cream and coconut oil into it.
2. Whisk using an electric beater.
3. Whisk until the mixture becomes smooth and glossy.
4. Add cocoa powder slowly and mix well.
5. Add in the rest of the ingredients.
6. Pour into a bread pan lined with parchment paper.
7. Freeze until set.
8. Cut them into squares and serve.

Nutrition (Per Serving)

- Total Carbs: 1g
- Fiber: 1g
- Protein: 0g
- Fat: 20g

No Bake Cheesecake

Serving: 10
Prep Time: 120 minutes
Cook Time: Nil
Ingredients:
For Crust

- 2 tablespoons ground flaxseeds
- 2 tablespoons desiccated coconut
- 1 teaspoon cinnamon

For Filling

- 4 ounces vegan cream cheese
- 1 cup cashews, soaked
- ½ cup frozen blueberries
- 2 tablespoons coconut oil
- 1 tablespoon lemon juice
- 1 teaspoon vanilla extract
- Liquid stevia

How To:

1. Take a container and mix in the crust ingredients, mix well.
2. Flatten the mixture at the bottom to prepare the crust of your cheesecake.
3. Take a blender/ food processor and add the filling ingredients, blend until smooth.
4. Gently pour the batter on top of your crust and chill for 2 hours.
5. Serve and enjoy!

Nutrition (Per Serving)

- Calories: 182
- Fat: 16g
- Carbohydrates: 4g
- Protein: 3g

Easy Chia Seed Pumpkin Pudding

Serving: 4
Prep Time: 10-15 minutes/ overnight chill time
Cook Time: Nil
Ingredients:

- 1 cup maple syrup
- 2 teaspoons pumpkin spice
- 1 cup pumpkin puree
- 1 ¼ cup almond milk
- ½ cup chia seeds

How To:

1. Add all of the ingredients to a bowl and gently stir.
2. Let it refrigerate overnight or at least 15 minutes.
3. Top with your desired ingredients, such as blueberries, almonds, etc.
4. Serve and enjoy!

Nutrition (Per Serving)

- Calories: 230
- Fat: 10g
- Carbohydrates:22g
- Protein:11g

Lovely Blueberry Pudding

Serving: 4
Prep Time: 20 minutes
Cook Time: Nil
Smart Points: 0
Ingredients:

- 2 cups frozen blueberries
- 2 teaspoons lime zest, grated freshly
- 20 drops liquid stevia
- 2 small avocados, peeled, pitted and chopped
- ½ teaspoon fresh ginger, grated freshly
- 4 tablespoons fresh lime juice
- 10 tablespoons water

How To:

1. Add all of the listed ingredients to a blender (except blueberries) and pulse the mixture well.
2. Transfer the mix into small serving bowls and chill the bowls.
3. Serve with a topping of blueberries.
4. Enjoy!

Nutrition (Per Serving)

- Calories: 166
- Fat: 13g
- Carbohydrates: 13g
- Protein: 1.7g

Decisive Lime and Strawberry Popsicle

Serving: 4
Prep Time: 2 hours
Cook Time: Nil
Ingredients:

- 1 tablespoon lime juice, fresh
- ¼ cup strawberries, hulled and sliced
- ¼ cup coconut almond milk, unsweetened and full fat
- 2 teaspoons natural sweetener

How To:

1. Blend the listed ingredients in a blender until smooth.
2. Pour mix into popsicle molds and let them chill for 2 hours.
3. Serve and enjoy!

Nutrition (Per Serving)

- Calories: 166
- Fat: 17g
- Carbohydrates: 3g
- Protein: 1g

Ravaging Blueberry Muffin

Serving: 4
Prep Time: 10 minutes
Cook Time: 30 minutes
Ingredients:

- 1 cup almond flour
- Pinch of sunflower seeds
- 1/8 teaspoon baking soda
- 1 whole egg
- 2 tablespoons coconut oil, melted
- ½ cup coconut almond milk
- ¼ cup fresh blueberries

How To:

1. Pre-heat your oven to 350 degrees F.
2. Line a muffin tin with paper muffin cups.
3. Add almond flour, sunflower seeds, baking soda to a bowl and mix, keep it on the side.
4. Take another bowl and add egg, coconut oil, coconut almond milk and mix.
5. Add mix to flour mix and gently combine until incorporated.
6. Mix in blueberries and fill the cupcakes tins with batter.
7. Bake for 20-25 minutes.
8. Enjoy!

Nutrition (Per Serving)

- Calories: 167
- Fat: 15g
- Carbohydrates: 2.1g
- Protein: 5.2g

The Coconut Loaf

Serving: 4
Prep Time: 15 minutes
Cook Time: 40 minutes
Ingredients:

- 1 ½ tablespoons coconut flour
- ¼ teaspoon baking powder
- 1/8 teaspoon sunflower seeds
- 1 tablespoons coconut oil, melted
- 1 whole egg

How To:

1. Pre-heat your oven to 350 degrees F.
2. Add coconut flour, baking powder, sunflower seeds.
3. Add coconut oil, eggs and stir well until mixed.
4. Leave batter for several minutes.
5. Pour half batter onto baking pan.
6. Spread it to form a circle, repeat with remaining batter.
7. Bake in oven for 10 minutes.
8. Once you have a golden brown texture, let it cool and serve.
9. Enjoy!

Nutrition (Per Serving)

- Calories: 297
- Fat: 14g
- Carbohydrates: 15g
- Protein: 15g

Fresh Figs with Walnuts and Ricotta

Serving: 4
Prep Time: 5 minutes
Cook Time: 2-3 minutes
Ingredients:

- 8 dried figs, halved
- ¼ cup ricotta cheese
- 16 walnuts, halved
- 1 tablespoon honey

How To:

1. Take a skillet and place it over medium heat, add walnuts and toast for 2 minutes.
2. Top figs with cheese and walnuts.
3. Drizzle honey on top.
4. Enjoy!

Nutrition (Per Serving)

- Calories: 142
- Fat: 8g
- Carbohydrates:10g
- Protein:4g

Authentic Medjool Date Truffles

Serving: 4
Prep Time: 10-15 minutes
Cook Time: Nil
Ingredients:

- 2 tablespoons peanut oil
- ½ cup popcorn kernels
- 1/3 cup peanuts, chopped
- 1/3 cup peanut almond butter
- ¼ cup wildflower honey

How To:

1. Take a pot and add popcorn kernels, peanut oil.
2. Place it over medium heat and shake the pot gently until all corn has popped.
3. Take a saucepan and add honey, gently simmer for 2-3 minutes.
4. Add peanut almond butter and stir.
5. Coat popcorn with the mixture and enjoy!

Nutrition (Per Serving)

- Calories: 430
- Fat: 20g
- Carbohydrates: 56g
- Protein 9g

Tasty Mediterranean Peanut Almond butter Popcorns

Serving: 4
Prep Time: 5 minutes + 20 minutes chill time
Cook Time: 2-3 minutes
Ingredients:

- 3 cups Medjool dates, chopped
- 12 ounces brewed coffee
- 1 cup pecans, chopped
- ½ cup coconut, shredded
- ½ cup cocoa powder

How To:

1. Soak dates in warm coffee for 5 minutes.
2. Remove dates from coffee and mash them, making a fine smooth mixture.
3. Stir in remaining ingredients (except cocoa powder) and form small balls out of the mixture.
4. Coat with cocoa powder, serve and enjoy!

Nutrition (Per Serving)

- Calories: 265
- Fat: 12g
- Carbohydrates: 43g
- Protein 3g

Just A Minute Worth Muffin

Serving: 2
Prep Time: 5 minutes
Cooking Time: 1 minute
Ingredients:

- Coconut oil for grease
- 2 teaspoons coconut flour
- 1 pinch baking soda
- 1 pinch sunflower seeds
- 1 whole egg

How To:

1. Grease ramekin dish with coconut oil and keep it on the side.
2. Add ingredients to a bowl and combine until no lumps.
3. Pour batter into ramekin.
4. Microwave for 1 minute on HIGH.
5. Slice in half and serve.
6. Enjoy!

Nutrition (Per Serving)

- Total Carbs: 5.4
- Fiber: 2g
- Protein: 7.3g

Hearty Almond Bread

Serving: 8
Prep Time: 15 minutes
Cook Time: 60 minutes
Ingredients:

- 3 cups almond flour
- 1 teaspoon baking soda
- 2 teaspoons baking powder
- ¼ teaspoon sunflower seeds
- ¼ cup almond milk
- ½ cup + 2 tablespoons olive oil
- 3 whole eggs

How To:

1. Pre-heat your oven to 300 degrees F.
2. Take a 9x5 inch loaf pan and grease, keep it on the side.
3. Add listed ingredients to a bowl and pour the batter into the loaf pan.
4. Bake for 60 minutes.
5. Once baked, remove from oven and let it cool.
6. Slice and serve!

Nutrition (Per Serving)

- Calories: 277
- Fat: 21g
- Carbohydrates: 7g
- Protein: 10g

Chapter 5: Smoothies and Drinks Recipes

Mixed Berries Smoothie

Serving: 2
Prep Time: 4 minutes
Cook Time: 0 minutes

Ingredients:

- ¼ cup frozen blueberries
- ¼ cup frozen blackberries
- 1 cup unsweetened almond milk
- 1 teaspoon vanilla bean extract
- 3 teaspoons flaxseeds
- 1 scoop chilled Greek yogurt
- Stevia as needed

How To:

1. Mix everything in a blender and emulsify.
2. Pulse the mixture four time until you have your desired thickness.
3. Pour the mixture into a glass and enjoy!

Nutrition (Per Serving)

- Calories: 221
- Fat: 9g
- Protein: 21g
- Carbohydrates: 10g

Satisfying Berry and Almond Smoothie

Serving: 4
Prep Time: 10 minutes
Cook Time: nil

Ingredients:

- 1 cup blueberries, frozen
- 1 whole banana
- ½ cup almond milk
- 1 tablespoon almond butter
- Water as needed

How To:

1. Add the listed ingredients to your blender and blend well until you have a smoothie-like texture.
2. Chill and serve.
3. Enjoy!

Nutrition (Per Serving)

- Calories: 321
- Fat: 11g
- Carbohydrates: 55g
- Protein: 5g

Refreshing Mango and Pear Smoothie

Serving: 1
Prep Time: 10 minutes
Cook Time: Nil
Ingredients:

- 1 ripe mango, cored and chopped
- ½ mango, peeled, pitted and chopped
- 1 cup kale, chopped
- ½ cup plain Greek yogurt
- 2 ice cubes

How To:

1. Add pear, mango, yogurt, kale, and mango to a blender and puree.

2. Add ice and blend until you have a smooth texture.

3. Serve and enjoy!

Nutrition (Per Serving)

- Calories: 293
- Fat: 8g
- Carbohydrates: 53g
- Protein: 8g

Epic Pineapple Juice

Serving: 4
Prep Time: 10 minutes
Cook Time: nil
Ingredients:

- 4 cups fresh pineapple, chopped
- 1 pinch sunflower seeds
- 1 ½ cups water

How To:

1. Add the listed ingredients to your blender and blend well until you have a smoothie-like texture.
2. Chill and serve.
3. Enjoy!

Nutrition (Per Serving)

- Calories: 82
- Fat: 0.2g
- Carbohydrates: 21g
- Protein: 21

Choco Lovers Strawberry Shake

Serving: 1
Prep Time: 10 minutes
Ingredients:
- ½ cup heavy cream, liquid
- 1 tablespoons cocoa powder
- 1 pack stevia
- ½ cup strawberry, sliced
- 1 tablespoon coconut flakes, unsweetened
- 1 ½ cups water

How To:
1. Add listed ingredients to blender.
2. Blend until you have a smooth and creamy texture.
3. Serve chilled and enjoy!

Nutrition (Per Serving)
- Calories: 470
- Fat: 46g
- Carbohydrates: 15g
- Protein: 4g

Healthy Coffee Smoothie

Serving: 1
Prep Time: 10 minutes
Ingredients:
- 1 tablespoon chia seeds
- 2 cups stongly brewed coffee, chilled
- 1 ounce Macadamia Nuts
- 1-2 packets stevia, optional
- 1 tablespoon MCT oil

How To:
1. Add all the listed ingredients to a blender.
2. Blend on high until smooth and creamy.
3. Enjoy your smoothie.

Nutrition (Per Serving)
- Calories: 395
- Fat: 39g
- Carbohydrates: 11g
- Protein: 5.2g

Blackberry and Apple Smoothie

Serving: 2
Prep Time: 5 minutes
Ingredients:

- 2 cups frozen blackberries
- ½ cup apple cider
- 1 apple, cubed
- 2/3 cup non-fat lemon yogurt

How To:

1. Add the listed ingredients to your blender and blend until smooth.
2. Serve chilled!

Nutrition (Per Serving)

- Calories: 200
- Fat: 10g
- Carbohydrates: 14g
- Protein 2g

The Mean Green Smoothie

Serving: 2
Prep Time: 5 minutes
Ingredients:

- 1 avocado
- 1 handful spinach, chopped
- Cucumber, 2 inch slices, peeled
- 1 lime, chopped
- Handful of grapes, chopped
- 5 dates, stoned and chopped
- 1 cup apple juice (fresh)

How To:

1. Add all the listed ingredients to your blender.
2. Blend until smooth.
3. Add a few ice cubes and serve the smoothie.
4. Enjoy!

Nutrition (Per Serving)

- Calories: 200
- Fat: 10g
- Carbohydrates: 14g
- Protein 2g

Mint Flavored Pear Smoothie

Serving: 2
Prep Time: 5 minutes
Ingredients:

- ¼ honey dew
- 2 green pears, ripe
- ½ apple, juiced
- 1 cup ice cubes
- ½ cup fresh mint leaves

How To:
1. Add the listed ingredients to your blender and blend until smooth.
2. Serve chilled!
Nutrition (Per Serving)

- Calories: 200
- Fat: 10g
- Carbohydrates: 14g
- Protein 2g

Chilled Watermelon Smoothie

Serving: 2
Prep Time: 5 minutes
Ingredients:

- 1 cup watermelon chunks
- ½ cup coconut water
- 1 ½ teaspoons lime juice
- 4 mint leaves
- 4 ice cubes

How To:
1. Add the listed ingredients to your blender and blend until smooth.
2. Serve chilled!
Nutrition (Per Serving)

- Calories: 200
- Fat: 10g
- Carbohydrates: 14g
- Protein 2g

Banana Ginger Medley

Serving: 2
Prep Time: 5 minutes
Ingredients:

- 1 banana, sliced
- ¾ cup vanilla yogurt
- 1 tablespoon honey
- ½ teaspoon ginger, grated

How To:

1. Add the listed ingredients to your blender and blend until smooth.
2. Serve chilled!

Nutrition (Per Serving)

- Calories: 200
- Fat: 10g
- Carbohydrates: 14g
- Protein 2g

Banana and Almond Flax Glass

Serving: 2
Prep Time: 5 minutes
Ingredients:

- 1 ripe frozen banana, diced
- 2/3 cup unsweetened almond milk
- 1/3 cup fat free plain Greek Yogurt
- 1 ½ tablespoons almond butter
- 1 tablespoon flaxseed meal
- 1 teaspoon honey
- 2-3 drops almond extract

How To:

1. Add the listed ingredients to your blender and blend until smooth
2. Serve chilled!

Nutrition (Per Serving)

- Calories: 200
- Fat: 10g
- Carbohydrates: 14g
- Protein 2g

Sensational Strawberry Medley

Serving: 2
Prep Time: 5 minutes
Ingredients:

- 1-2 handful baby greens
- 3 medium kale leaves
- 5-8 mint leaves
- 1 inch piece ginger , peeled
- 1 avocado
- 1 cup strawberries
- 6-8 ounces coconut water + 6-8 ounces filtered water
- Fresh juice of one lime
- 1-2 teaspoon olive oil

How To:

1. Add all the listed ingredients to your blender.
2. Blend until smooth.
3. Add a few ice cubes and serve the smoothie.
4. Enjoy!

Nutrition (Per Serving)

- Calories: 200
- Fat: 10g
- Carbohydrates: 14g
- Protein 2g

Mango's Gone Haywire

Serving: 2
Prep Time: 5 minutes
Ingredients:

- 1 mango, diced
- 2 bananas, diced
- 1-2 oranges, quartered
- Dash of lemon juice
- 1 tablespoon hemp seed
- ¼ teaspoon green powder
- Coconut water (as needed)

How To:

1. Add orange quarters in the blender first, blend.
2. Add the remaining ingredients and blend until smooth.
3. Add more coconut water to adjust the thickness.
4. Serve chilled!

Nutrition (Per Serving)

- Calories: 200
- Fat: 10g
- Carbohydrates: 14g
- Protein 2g

Unexpectedly Awesome Orange Smoothie

Serving: 2
Prep Time: 5 minutes
Ingredients:

- 1 orange, peeled
- ¼ cup fat-free yogurt
- 2 tablespoons frozen orange juice concentrate
- ¼ teaspoon vanilla extract
- 4 ice cubes

How To:

1. Add the listed ingredients to your blender and blend until smooth.
2. Serve chilled!

Nutrition (Per Serving)

- Calories: 200
- Fat: 10g
- Carbohydrates: 14g
- Protein 2g

Minty Cherry Smoothie

Serving: 2
Prep Time: 5 minutes
Ingredients:

- ¾ cup cherries
- 1 teaspoon mint
- ½ cup almond milk
- ½ cup kale
- ½ teaspoon fresh vanilla

How To:

1. Wash and cut cherries.
2. Take the pits out.
3. Add cherries to blender.
4. Pour almond milk.
5. Wash the mint and put two sprigs in the blender.
6. Separate the kale leaves from the stems.
7. Put kale in blender.
8. Press vanilla bean and cut lengthwise with knife.
9. Scoop out your desired amount of vanilla and add to the blender.
10. Blend until smooth.
11. Serve chilled and enjoy!

Nutrition (Per Serving)

- Calories: 200
- Fat: 10g
- Carbohydrates: 14g
- Protein 2g

A Very Berry (and Green) Smoothie

Serving: 2
Prep Time: 5 minutes
Ingredients:

- 1 cup spinach leaves
- ½ cup frozen blueberries
- 1 ripe banana
- ½ cup milk
- 2 tablespoons old fashioned oats
- ½ tablespoon stevia

How To:
1. Add the listed ingredients to your blender and blend until smooth.
2. Serve chilled!

Nutrition (Per Serving)

- Calories: 200
- Fat: 10g
- Carbohydrates: 14g
- Protein 2g

Authentic Ginger and Berry Smoothie

Serving: 2
Prep Time: 5 minutes
Cook Time: Nil
Ingredients:

- 2 cups blackberries
- 2 cups unsweetened almond milk
- 1 -2 packs of stevia
- 1 piece of 1-inch fresh ginger, peeled and roughly chopped
- 2 cups crushed ice

How To:
1. Add the listed ingredients to a blender and blend the whole mixture until smooth.
2. Serve chilled and enjoy!

Nutrition (Per Serving)

- Calories: 200
- Fat: 10g
- Carbohydrates: 14g
- Protein 2g

A Glassful of Kale and Spinach

Serving: 2
Prep Time: 5 minutes
Ingredients:

- Handful of kale
- Handful of spinach
- 2 broccoli heads
- 1 tomato
- Handful of lettuce
- 1 avocado, cubed
- 1 cucumber, cubed
- Juice of ½ lemon
- Pineapple juice as needed

How To:

1. Add all the listed ingredients to your blender.
2. Blend until smooth.
3. Add a few ice cubes and serve the smoothie.
4. Enjoy!

Nutrition (Per Serving)

- Calories: 200
- Fat: 10g
- Carbohydrates: 14g
- Protein 2g

Green Tea, Turmeric, and Mango Smoothie

Serving: 2
Prep Time: 5 minutes
Ingredients:

- 2 cups mango, cubed
- 2 teaspoons turmeric powder
- 2 tablespoons Green Tea powder
- 2 cups almond milk
- 2 tablespoons honey
- 1 cup crushed ice

How To:

1. Add the listed ingredients to a blender and blend the whole mixture until smooth.
2. Serve chilled and enjoy!

Nutrition (Per Serving)

- Calories: 200
- Fat: 10g
- Carbohydrates: 14g
- Protein 2g

The Great Anti-Oxidant Glass

Serving: 2
Prep Time: 5 minutes
Ingredients:

- 1 whole ripe avocado
- 4 cups organic baby spinach leaves
- 1 cup filtered water
- Juice of 1 lemon
- 1 English cucumber, chopped
- 3 stems fresh parsley
- 5 stems fresh mint
- 1-inch piece fresh ginger
- 2 large ice cubes

How To:

1. Add all the listed ingredients to your blender.
2. Blend until smooth.
3. Add a few ice cubes and serve the smoothie.
4. Enjoy!

Nutrition (Per Serving)

- Calories: 200
- Fat: 10g
- Carbohydrates: 14g
- Protein 2g

Fresh Minty Smoothie

Serving: 1
Prep Time: 10 minutes
Ingredients:

- 1 stalk celery
- 2 cups water
- 2 ounces almonds
- 1 packet stevia
- 1 cup spinach
- 2 mint leaves

How To:

1. Add listed ingredients to blender.
2. Blend until you have a smooth and creamy texture.
3. Serve chilled and enjoy!

Nutrition (Per Serving)

- Calories: 417
- Fat: 43g
- Carbohydrates: 10g
- Protein: 5.5g

Refreshing Mango and Pear Smoothie

Serving: 1
Prep Time: 10 minutes
Cook Time: Nil
Ingredients:

- 1 ripe mango, cored and chopped
- ½ mango, peeled, pitted and chopped
- 1 cup kale, chopped
- ½ cup plain Greek yogurt
- 2 ice cubes

How To:

1. Add pear, mango, yogurt, kale, and mango to a blender and puree.
2. Add ice and blend until you have a smooth texture.
3. Serve and enjoy!

Nutrition (Per Serving)

- Calories: 293
- Fat: 8g
- Carbohydrates: 53g
- Protein: 8g

Coconut and Hazelnut Chilled Glass

Serving: 1
Prep Time: 10 minutes
Ingredients:

- ½ cup coconut almond milk
- ¼ cup hazelnuts, chopped
- 1 ½ cups water
- 1 pack stevia

How To:

1. Add listed ingredients to blender.
2. Blend until you have a smooth and creamy texture.
3. Serve chilled and enjoy!

Nutrition (Per Serving)

- Calories: 457
- Fat: 46g
- Carbohydrates: 12g
- Protein: 7g

The Mocha Shake

Serving: 1
Prep Time: 10 minutes
Ingredients:
- 1 cup whole almond milk
- 2 tablespoons cocoa powder
- 2 packs stevia
- 1 cup brewed coffee, chilled
- 1 tablespoon coconut oil

How To:
1. Add listed ingredients to blender.
2. Blend until you have a smooth and creamy texture.
3. Serve chilled and enjoy!

Nutrition (Per Serving)
- Calories: 293
- Fat: 23g
- Carbohydrates: 19g
- Protein: 10g

Cinnamon Chiller

Serving: 1
Prep Time: 10 minutes
Ingredients:
- 1 cup unsweetened almond milk
- 2 tablespoons vanilla protein powder
- ½ teaspoon cinnamon
- ¼ teaspoon vanilla extract
- 1 tablespoon chia seeds
- 1 cup ice cubs

How To:
1. Add listed ingredients to blender.
2. Blend until you have a smooth and creamy texture.
3. Serve chilled and enjoy!

Nutrition (Per Serving)
- Calories: 145
- Fat: 4g
- Carbohydrates: 1.6g
- Protein: 0.6g

Hearty Alkaline Strawberry Summer Deluxe

Serving: 2
Prep Time: 5 minutes
Ingredients:

- ½ cup organic strawberries/blueberries
- Half a banana
- 2 cups coconut water
- ½ inch ginger
- Juice of 2 grapefruits

How To:

1. Add all the listed ingredients to your blender.
2. Blend until smooth.
3. Add a few ice cubes and serve the smoothie.
4. Enjoy!

Nutrition (Per Serving)

- Calories: 200
- Fat: 10g
- Carbohydrates: 14g
- Protein 2g

Delish Pineapple and Coconut Milk Smoothie

Serving: 2
Prep Time: 5 minutes
Ingredients:

- ¼ cup pineapple, frozen
- ¾ cup coconut milk

How To:

1. Add the listed ingredients to blender and blend well on high.
2. Once the mixture is smooth, pour smoothie in tall glass and serve.
3. Chill and enjoy!

Nutrition (Per Serving)

- Calories: 200
- Fat: 10g
- Carbohydrates: 14g
- Protein 2g

The Minty Refresher

Serving: 2
Prep Time: 5 minutes
Ingredients:

- 2 cups mint tea
- 1 cucumber, peeled
- 2 green apples
- 1 cup blueberries
- Stevia (to sweeten)
- Few slices of lime/lemon for garnish

How To:

1. Add the listed ingredients to your blender and blend until smooth.
2. Add ice and sweeten with a bit of stevia.
3. Garnish with lime/lemon slices.
4. Serve and enjoy!

Nutrition (Per Serving)

- Calories: 200
- Fat: 10g
- Carbohydrates: 14g
- Protein 2g

The "Upbeat" Strawberry and Clementine Glass

Serving: 2
Prep Time: 5 minutes
Ingredients:

- 8 ounces strawberries, fresh
- 1 banana, chopped into chunks
- 2 Clementines/Mandarins

How To:

1. Peel the clementines and remove seeds.
2. Add the listed ingredients to your blender/food processor and blend until smooth.
3. Serve chilled and enjoy!

Nutrition (Per Serving)

- Calories: 200
- Fat: 10g
- Carbohydrates: 14g
- Protein 2g

Cabbage and Coconut Chia Smoothie

Serving: 2
Prep Time: 5 minutes
Ingredients:

- 1/3 cup cabbage
- 1 cup cold unsweetened coconut milk
- 1 tablespoon chia seeds
- ½ cup cherries
- ½ cup spinach

How To:

1. Add coconut milk to your blender.
2. Cut cabbage and add to your blender.
3. Place chia seeds in a coffee grinder and chop to powder, brush the powder into the blender.
4. Pit the cherries and add them to the blender.
5. Wash and dry the spinach and chop.
6. Add to the mix.
7. Cover and blend on low followed by medium.
8. Taste the texture and serve chilled!

Nutrition (Per Serving)

- Calories: 200
- Fat: 10g
- Carbohydrates: 14g
- Protein 2g

The Cherry Beet Delight

Serving: 2
Prep Time: 5 minutes
Ingredients:

- 1 cup cherries, pitted
- ½ cup beets
- Few banana slices
- 1 cup water, filtered, alkaline
- 1 cup coconut milk
- Pinch of organic vanilla powder
- Pinch of cinnamon
- Pinch of stevia
- Few mint leaves/lime slices to garnish

How To:

1. Add berries, beets, water, banana slices, coconut milk to your blender.
2. Blend well until smooth.
3. Add more water if the texture is too creamy for you.
4. Add coconut oil, vanilla, cinnamon and stir.
5. Add a bit of stevia for extra sweetness.
6. Garnish with mint leaves and lime slices.
7. Enjoy!

Nutrition (Per Serving)

- Calories: 200
- Fat: 10g
- Carbohydrates: 14g
- Protein 2g

Green Delight

Serving: 1
Prep Time: 10 minutes
Ingredients:

- ¾ cup whole almond milk yogurt
- 2 ½ cups lettuce mix salad greens
- 1 pack stevia
- 1 tablespoon MCT oil
- 1 tablespoon chia seeds
- 1 ½ cups water

How To:

1. Add listed ingredients to blender.

2. Blend until you have a smooth and creamy texture.

3. Serve chilled and enjoy!

Nutrition (Per Serving)

- Calories: 320
- Fat: 24g
- Carbohydrates: 17g
- Protein: 10g

Guilt Free Lemon and Rosemary Drink

Serving: 1
Prep Time: 10 minutes
Ingredients:

- ½ cup whole almond milk yogurt
- 1 cup garden greens
- 1 pack stevia
- 1 tablespoon olive oil
- 1 stalk fresh rosemary

- 1 tablespoon lemon juice, fresh
- 1 tablespoon pepitas
- 1 tablespoon flaxseed, ground
- 1 ½ cups water

How To:
1. Add listed ingredients to blender.
2. Blend until you have a smooth and creamy texture.
3. Serve chilled and enjoy!

Nutrition (Per Serving)

- Calories: 312
- Fat: 25g

- Carbohydrates: 14g
- Protein: 9g

Strawberry and Rhubarb Smoothie

Serving: 1
Prep Time: 5 minutes
Cook Time: 3 minutes
Ingredients:

- 1 rhubarb stalk, chopped
- 1 cup fresh strawberries, sliced
- ½ cup plain Greek strawberries

- Pinch of ground cinnamon
- 3 ice cubes

How To:
1. Take a small saucepan and fill with water over high heat.
2. Bring to boil and add rhubarb, boil for 3 minutes.
3. Drain and transfer to a blender.
4. Add strawberries, honey, yogurt, cinnamon and pulse mixture until smooth.
5. Add ice cubes and blend until thick with no lumps.
6. Pour into glass and enjoy chilled.

Nutrition (Per Serving)

- Calories: 295
- Fat: 8g

- Carbohydrates: 56g
- Protein: 6g

Vanilla Hemp Drink

Serving: 1
Prep Time: 10 minutes
Ingredients:

- 1 cup water
- 1 cup unsweetened hemp almond milk, vanilla
- 1 ½ tablespoons coconut oil, unrefined
- ½ cup frozen blueberries, mixed
- 4 cups leafy greens, kale and spinach
- 1 tablespoon flaxseeds
- 1 tablespoon almond butter

How To:
1. Add listed ingredients to blender.
2. Blend until you have a smooth and creamy texture.
3. Serve chilled and enjoy!

Nutrition (Per Serving)

- Calories: 250
- Fat: 20g
- Carbohydrates: 10g
- Protein: 7g

Yogurt and Kale Smoothie

Serving: 1
Prep Time: 10 minutes
Ingredients:

- 1 cup whole almond milk yogurt
- 1 cup baby kale greens
- 1 pack stevia
- 1 tablespoon MCT oil
- 1 tablespoons sunflower seeds
- 1 cup water

How To:
1. Add listed ingredients to blender
2. Blend until you have a smooth and creamy texture
3. Serve chilled and enjoy!

Nutrition (Per Serving)

- Calories: 329
- Fat: 26g
- Carbohydrates: 15g
- Protein: 11g

The Sweet Potato Acid Buster

Serving: 2
Prep Time: 5 minutes
Ingredients:

- 1 cup sweet potato, chopped
- 1 cup almond milk
- ¼ teaspoon nutmeg
- ¼ teaspoon ground cinnamon

- 1 teaspoon flaxseed
- 1 small avocado, cubed
- Few spinach leaves, torn

Toppings:

- Handful of crushed almonds
- Handful of crushed cashews
- 3 tablespoons orange juice

How To:

1. Blend all the ingredients until smooth.
2. Add a few ice cubes to make it chilled.
3. Add your desired toppings.
4. Enjoy!

Nutrition (Per Serving)

- Calories: 200
- Fat: 10g

- Carbohydrates: 14g
- Protein 2g

The Sunshine Offering

Serving: 2
Prep Time: 5 minutes
Ingredients:

- 2 cups fresh spinach
- 1 ½ cups almond milk
- ½ cup coconut water

- 3 cups fresh pineapple
- 2 tablespoons coconut unsweetened flakes

How To:

1. Add all the listed ingredients to your blender.
2. Blend until smooth.
3. Add a few ice cubes and serve the smoothie.
4. Enjoy!

Nutrition (Per Serving)

- Calories: 200
- Fat: 10g

- Carbohydrates: 14g
- Protein 2g

The Sleepy Bug Smoothie

Serving: 2
Prep Time: 5 minutes
Ingredients:

- 1 cup fennel tea infusion
- 1 cup almond milk
- 1 cup watermelon, chopped
- 1 green apple
- ½ cup pomegranate
- ½ inch ginger
- Stevia to sweeten

How To:

1. Add the listed ingredients to your blender.
2. Blend until smooth.
3. Add a bit of stevia if you want more sweetness.
4. Serve chilled and enjoy!

Nutrition (Per Serving)

- Calories: 200
- Fat: 10g
- Carbohydrates: 14g
- Protein 2g

Matcha Coconut Smoothie

Serving: 2
Prep Time: 5 minutes
Cook Time: Nil
Ingredients:

- 1 whole banana, cubed
- 1 cup frozen mango, chunked
- 2 kale leaves, torn
- 3 tablespoons white beans
- 2 tablespoons shredded coconut
- ½ teaspoon Matcha green tea powder
- 1 cup water

How To:

1. Add banana, kale, mango, white beans, Matcha powder and white beans to the blender.
2. Blend until you have a nice smoothie.
3. Serve and enjoy!

Nutrition (Per Serving)

- Calories: 200
- Fat: 10g
- Carbohydrates: 14g
- Protein 2g

Ravishing Apple and Cucumber Glass

Serving: 2
Prep Time: 5 minutes
Ingredients:

- 1 green apple
- 2 cucumbers, peeled
- 1 cup almond milk
- ½ cup coconut cream (raw and organic)
- Pinch of cinnamon and nutmeg (each)
- Pinch of Himalayan salt
- 1 tablespoon coconut oil

How To:

1. Add all the listed ingredients to your blender (except oil, spices and salt).
2. Blend until smooth.
3. Mix in coconut oil, spices and salt.
4. Stir and enjoy!

Nutrition (Per Serving)

- Calories: 200
- Fat: 10g
- Carbohydrates: 14g
- Protein 2g

Creative Winter Smoothie

Serving: 2
Prep Time: 5 minutes
Ingredients:

- 3 tomatoes, peeled
- 1 celery stalk
- 2 cloves garlic, peeled
- 1-inch ginger, peeled
- 1 cucumber, peeled
- Juice of 1 lemon
- 1 cup alkaline water
- Salt as needed
- Pepper as needed
- Pinch of turmeric
- Olive oil/avocado oil

How To:

1. Add tomatoes, celery, garlic, cucumber and water to your blender.
2. Blend well until smooth.
3. Add lemon juice, salt and oil.
4. Stir.
5. Season with pepper and turmeric.
6. Stir.
7. Serve chilled and enjoy!

Nutrition (Per Serving)

- Calories: 200
- Fat: 10g
- Carbohydrates: 14g
- Protein 2g

Feisty Mango and Coconut Smoothie

Serving: 2
Prep Time: 5 minutes
Ingredients:

- 1 teaspoon spirulina
- 1 cup frozen mango
- 1 cup unsweetened coconut milk
- ½ cup spinach

How To:

1. Cut mangoes and dice them.
2. Add mango, cup of unsweetened coconut milk, teaspoon of Spirulina and spinach to the blender.
3. Blend on low to medium until smooth.
4. Check the texture and serve chilled!

Nutrition (Per Serving)

- Calories: 200
- Fat: 10g
- Carbohydrates: 14g
- Protein 2g

Mexican Chocolate Stand-Off

Serving: 2
Prep Time: 5 minutes
Ingredients:

- 2 bananas
- 1 tablespoon hemp seeds
- 1 bag frozen blueberries
- ½ teaspoon liquid stevia
- Pure water
- 2 teaspoons raw chocolate
- 1 teaspoon raw carob powder
- ½ teaspoon green powder
- ½ teaspoon cinnamon powder
- Pinch of cayenne pepper

How To:

1. Add all the listed ingredients to your blender.
2. Blend until smooth.
3. Add a few ice cubes and serve the smoothie.
4. Enjoy!

Nutrition (Per Serving)

- Calories: 200
- Fat: 10g
- Carbohydrates: 14g
- Protein 2g

The Awesome Cleanser

Serving: 2
Prep Time: 5 minutes
Ingredients:

- 2 grapefruits, juiced
- 2 lemons, juiced
- Half cup alkaline water/filtered water
- 2 tablespoons olive oil
- 2 cucumbers, peeled
- 1 avocado, peeled and pitted
- 2 cloves fresh garlic
- 1-inch ginger
- Pinch of Himalayan salt
- Pinch of cayenne pepper

How To:

1. Add cucumber, ginger, avocado, grapefruit and lemon to your blender.
2. Blend until smooth.
3. Add alkaline water, spices and oil.
4. Stir well and drink chilled.
5. Enjoy!

Nutrition (Per Serving)

- Calories: 200
- Fat: 10g
- Carbohydrates: 14g
- Protein 2g

Gentle Tropical Papaya Smoothie

Serving: 2
Prep Time: 5 minutes
Ingredients:

- 1 papaya, cut into chunks
- 1 cup fat free plain yogurt
- ½ cup pineapple chunks
- ½ cup crushed ice
- 1 teaspoon coconut extract
- 1 teaspoon flaxseed

How To:

1. Add the listed ingredients to your blender and blend until smooth.
2. Serve chilled!

Nutrition (Per Serving)

- Calories: 200
- Fat: 10g
- Carbohydrates: 14g
- Protein 2g

Kale and Apple Smoothie

Serving: 2
Prep Time: 5 minutes
Ingredients:

- ¾ of a kale, chopped, ribs and stem removed
- 1 small stalk celery, chopped
- ½ banana
- ½ cup apple juice
- 1 tablespoon lemon juice

How To:
1. Add the listed ingredients to your blender and blend until smooth.
2. Serve chilled!

Nutrition (Per Serving)

- Calories: 200
- Fat: 10g
- Carbohydrates: 14g
- Protein 2g

Mango and Lime Generous Smoothie

Serving: 2
Prep Time: 5 minutes
Ingredients:

- 2 tablespoons lime juice
- 2 cups spinach, chopped and stemmed
- 1 ½ cups frozen mango, cubed
- 1 cup green grapes

How To:
1. Add the listed ingredients to your blender and blend until smooth
2. Serve chilled!

Nutrition (Per Serving)

- Calories: 200
- Fat: 10g
- Carbohydrates: 14g
- Protein 2g

The Pear and Chocolate Catastrophe

Serving: 2
Prep Time: 5 minutes
Ingredients:

- 1 banana (freckled skin)
- 2-3 pears
- 2 tablespoons hulled hemp seeds
- 1 bag frozen raspberries
- 2 ½ cups coconut water
- 1 teaspoon raw chocolate
- Small bunch arugula lettuce leaves
- Liquid stevia

How To:

1. Add all the listed ingredients to your blender.
2. Blend until smooth.
3. Add a few ice cubes and serve the smoothie.
4. Enjoy!

Nutrition (Per Serving)

- Calories: 200
- Fat: 10g
- Carbohydrates: 14g
- Protein 2g

The Avocado Paradise

Serving: 2
Prep Time: 5 minutes
Ingredients:

- ½ avocado, cubed
- 1 cup coconut milk
- Half a lemon
- ¼ cup fresh spinach leaves
- 1 pear
- 1 tablespoon hemp seed powder

Toppings:

- Handful of macadamia nuts
- Handful of grapes
- 2 lemon slices

How To:

1. Blend all the ingredients until smooth.
2. Add a few ice cubes to make it chilled.
3. Add your desired toppings.
4. Enjoy!

Nutrition (Per Serving)

- Calories: 200
- Fat: 10g
- Carbohydrates: 14g
- Protein 2g

The Authentic Vegetable Medley

Serving: 2
Prep Time: 5 minutes
Ingredients:

- 1 cup broccoli, steamed
- 1 bunch asparagus, steamed
- 2 cups coconut milk
- 2 tablespoons coconut oil
- 2 carrots, peeled
- Few inches of horseradish
- Himalayan salt
- Pinch of chili powder
- ½ onion
- 2 garlic cloves

How To:

1. Add all the listed ingredients to your blender except coconut oil, salt and chili powder.
2. Blend until smooth.
3. Add salt, coconut oil and chili powder.
4. Stir well and serve chilled!

Nutrition (Per Serving)

- Calories: 200
- Fat: 10g
- Carbohydrates: 14g
- Protein 2g

The Original Power Producer

Serving: 2
Prep Time: 5 minutes
Ingredients:

- ½ cup spinach
- 1 avocado, diced
- 1 cup coconut milk
- 1 tablespoon flaxseed
- 2 nori sheets, roasted and crushed
- 1 garlic clove
- Salt to taste

Toppings:

- Handful of pistachios
- 3 tablespoons bell pepper, finely chopped
- Handful of parsley leaves

How To:

1. Blend all the ingredients until smooth.
2. Add a few ice cubes to make it chilled.
3. Add your desired toppings.
4. Enjoy!

Nutrition (Per Serving)

- Calories: 200
- Fat: 10g
- Carbohydrates: 14g
- Protein 2g

The Dreamy Cherry Mix

Serving: 2
Prep Time: 5 minutes
Ingredients:

- ½ cup ripe cherries
- Juice of 1 lemon
- 1 cup coconut milk
- 1 avocado, cubed
- ¼ cup spinach
- Few slices of cucumber, peeled

Toppings:

- Handful of pistachios
- Handful of raisins
- 1 slice lemon

How To:

1. Blend all the ingredients until smooth.
2. Add a few ice cubes to make it chilled.
3. Add your desired toppings.
4. Enjoy!

Nutrition (Per Serving)

- Calories: 200
- Fat: 10g
- Carbohydrates: 14g
- Protein 2g

Better Than Your Favorite Restaurant "Lemon Smoothie"

Serving: 2
Prep Time: 5 minutes
Ingredients:

- 2 cups organic rice milk, gluten free
- 1 cup melon, chopped
- ½ avocado, cubed
- ½ cucumber, peeled and sliced
- Ice cubes
- 2 limes, juiced
- 1 tablespoon coconut oil
- Few banana slices to taste

How To:

1. Add the listed ingredients to your blender (except coconut oil) and blend well.
2. Blend until you have a smooth texture.
3. Add coconut oil and stir.
4. Enjoy!

Nutrition (Per Serving)

- Calories: 200
- Fat: 10g
- Carbohydrates: 14g
- Protein 2g

The "One" with The Watermelon

Serving: 2
Prep Time: 5 minutes
Ingredients:

- 1 cup watermelon, sliced
- ½ cup coconut, shredded
- 1 grapefruit, cubed
- ½ cup coconut milk
- 2 tablespoons almond butter

Toppings:

- Handful of crushed almonds
- Handful of raisins
- 2 tablespoons coconut powder

How To:

1. Blend all the ingredients until smooth.
2. Add a few ice cubes to make it chilled.
3. Add your desired toppings.
4. Enjoy!

Nutrition (Per Serving)

- Calories: 200
- Fat: 10g
- Carbohydrates: 14g
- Protein 2g

Strawberry and Rhubarb Smoothie

Serving: 1
Prep Time: 5 minutes
Cook Time: 3 minutes
Ingredients:

- 1 rhubarb stalk, chopped
- 1 cup fresh strawberries, sliced
- ½ cup plain Greek yoghurt
- Pinch of ground cinnamon
- 3 ice cubes

How To:

1. Take a small saucepan and fill with water over high heat.
2. Bring to boil and add rhubarb, boil for 3 minutes.
3. Drain and transfer to a blender.
4. Add strawberries, honey, yogurt, cinnamon and pulse mixture until smooth.
5. Add ice cubes and blend until thick and has no lumps.
6. Pour into glass and enjoy chilled.

Nutrition (Per Serving)

- Calories: 295
- Fat: 8g
- Carbohydrates: 56g
- Protein: 6g

Chapter 6: Vegetarian and Vegan Recipes

Spinach Dip

Serving: 2
Prep Time: 4 minutes
Cook Time: 0 minutes
Ingredients:

- 5 ounces Spinach, raw
- 1 cup Greek yogurt
- 1/2 tablespoon onion powder
- 1/4 teaspoon garlic sunflower seeds
- Black pepper to taste
- 1/4 teaspoon Greek Seasoning

How To:

1. Add the listed ingredients in a blender.
2. Emulsify.
3. Season and serve.

Nutrition (Per Serving)

- Calories: 101
- Fat: 4g
- Carbohydrates: 4g
- Protein: 10g

Cauliflower Rice

Serving: 2
Prep Time: 5 minutes
Cook Time: 6 minutes
Ingredients:

- 1 head grated cauliflower head
- 1 tablespoon coconut aminos
- 1 pinch of sunflower seeds
- 1 pinch of black pepper
- 1 tablespoon Garlic Powder
- 1 tablespoon Sesame Oil

How To:

1. Add cauliflower to a food processor and grate it.
2. Take a pan and add sesame oil, let it heat up over medium heat.
3. Add grated cauliflower and pour coconut aminos.
4. Cook for 4-6 minutes.
5. Season and enjoy!

Nutrition (Per Serving)

- Calories: 329
- Fat: 28g
- Carbohydrates: 13g
- Protein: 10g

Grilled Sprouts and Balsamic Glaze

Serving: 2
Prep Time: 10 minutes
Cook Time: 30 minutes
Smart Points: 4
Ingredients:

- ½ pound Brussels sprouts, trimmed and halved
- Fresh cracked black pepper
- 1 tablespoon olive oil
- Sunflower seeds to taste
- 2 teaspoons balsamic glaze
- 2 wooden skewers

How To:

1. Take wooden skewers and place them on a largely sized foil.
2. Place sprouts on the skewers and drizzle oil, sprinkle sunflower seeds and pepper.
3. Cover skewers with foil.
4. Pre-heat your grill to low and place skewers (with foil) in the grill.
5. Grill for 30 minutes, making sure to turn after every 5-6 minutes.
6. Once done, uncovered and drizzle balsamic glaze on top.
7. Enjoy!

Nutrition (Per Serving)

- Calories: 440
- Fat: 27g
- Carbohydrates: 33g
- Protein: 26g

Amazing Green Creamy Cabbage

Serving: 4
Prep Time: 10 minutes
Cook Time: 10 minutes
Ingredients:

- 2 ounces almond butter
- 1 ½ pounds green cabbage, shredded
- 1 ¼ cups coconut cream
- Sunflower seeds and pepper to taste
- 8 tablespoons fresh parsley, chopped

How To:

1. Take a skillet and place it over medium heat, add almond butter and let it melt.
2. Add cabbage and sauté until brown.
3. Stir in cream and lower the heat to low.
4. Let it simmer.
5. Season with sunflower seeds and pepper.
6. Garnish with parsley and serve.
7. Enjoy!

Nutrition (Per Serving)

- Calories: 432
- Fat: 42g
- Carbohydrates: 8g
- Protein: 4g

Simple Rice Mushroom Risotto

Serving: 4

Prep Time: 5 minutes

Cook Time: 15 minutes

Ingredients:

- 4 ½ cups cauliflower, riced
- 3 tablespoons coconut oil
- 1 pound Portobello mushrooms, thinly sliced
- 1 pound white mushrooms, thinly sliced
- 2 shallots, diced
- ¼ cup organic vegetable broth
- Sunflower seeds and pepper to taste
- 3 tablespoons chives, chopped
- 4 tablespoons almond butter
- ½ cup kite ricotta/cashew cheese, grated

How To:

1. Use a food processor and pulse cauliflower florets until riced.
2. Take a large saucepan and heat up 2 tablespoons oil over medium-high flame.
3. Add mushrooms and sauté for 3 minutes until mushrooms are tender.
4. Clear saucepan of mushrooms and liquid and keep them on the side.
5. Add the rest of the 1 tablespoon oil to skillet.
6. Toss shallots and cook for 60 seconds.
7. Add cauliflower rice, stir for 2 minutes until coated with oil.
8. Add broth to riced cauliflower and stir for 5 minutes.
9. Remove pot from heat and mix in mushrooms and liquid.
10. Add chives, almond butter, parmesan cheese.
11. Season with sunflower seeds and pepper.
12. Serve and enjoy!

Nutrition (Per Serving)

- Calories: 438
- Fat: 17g
- Carbohydrates: 15g
- Protein: 12g

Hearty Green Bean Roast

Serving: 4

Prep Time: 10 minutes

Cook Time: 20 minutes

Ingredients:

- 1 whole egg
- 2 tablespoons olive oil
- Sunflower seeds and pepper to taste
- 1 pound fresh green beans
- 5 ½ tablespoons grated parmesan cheese

How To:

1. Pre-heat your oven to 400 degrees F.
2. Take a bowl and whisk in eggs with oil and spices.
3. Add beans and mix well.
4. Stir in parmesan cheese and pour the mix into baking pan (lined with parchment paper).
5. Bake for 15-20 minutes.
6. Serve warm and enjoy!

Nutrition (Per Serving)

- Calories: 216
- Fat: 21g
- Carbohydrates: 7g
- Protein: 9g

Almond and Blistered Beans

Serving: 4
Prep Time: 10 minutes
Cook Time: 20 minutes
Ingredients:

- 1 pound fresh green beans, ends trimmed
- 1 ½ tablespoon olive oil
- ¼ teaspoon sunflower seeds
- 1 ½ tablespoons fresh dill, minced
- Juice of 1 lemon
- ¼ cup crushed almonds
- Sunflower seeds as needed

How To:

1. Pre-heat your oven to 400 degrees F.
2. Add the green beans with your olive oil and also the sunflower seeds.
3. Then spread them in one single layer on a large sized sheet pan.
4. Roast it for 10 minutes and stir, then roast for another 8-10 minutes.
5. Remove from the oven and keep stirring in the lemon juice alongside the dill.
6. Top it with crushed almonds and some flaked sunflower seeds and serve.

Nutrition (Per Serving)

- Calories: 347
- Fat: 16g
- Carbohydrates: 6g
- Protein: 45g

Tomato Platter

Serving: 8
Prep Time: 10 minutes + Chill time
Cook Time: Nil
Ingredients:

- 1/3 cup olive oil
- 1 teaspoon sunflower seeds
- 2 tablespoons onion, chopped
- ¼ teaspoon pepper
- ½ a garlic, minced
- 1 tablespoon fresh parsley, minced
- 3 large fresh tomatoes, sliced
- 1 teaspoon dried basil
- ¼ cup red wine vinegar

How To:

1. Take a shallow dish and arrange tomatoes in the dish.
2. Add the rest of the ingredients in a mason jar, cover the jar and shake it well.
3. Pour the mix over tomato slices.
4. Let it chill for 2-3 hours.
5. Serve!

Nutrition (Per Serving)

- Calories: 350
- Fat: 28g
- Carbohydrates: 10g
- Protein: 14g

Lemony Sprouts

Serving: 4
Prep Time: 10 minutes
Cook Time: Nil
Ingredients:

- 1 pound Brussels sprouts, trimmed and shredded
- 8 tablespoons olive oil
- 1 lemon, juice and zested
- Sunflower seeds and pepper to taste
- ¾ cup spicy almond and seed mix

How To:

1. Take a bowl and mix in lemon juice, sunflower seeds, pepper and olive oil.
2. Mix well.
3. Stir in shredded Brussels sprouts and toss.
4. Let it sit for 10 minutes.
5. Add nuts and toss.
6. Serve and enjoy!

Nutrition (Per Serving)

- Calories: 382
- Fat: 36g
- Carbohydrates: 9g
- Protein: 7g

Cool Garbanzo and Spinach Beans

Serving: 4
Prep Time: 5-10 minutes
Cook Time: Nil
Ingredients:

- 1 tablespoon olive oil
- ½ onion, diced
- 10 ounces spinach, chopped
- 12 ounces garbanzo beans
- ½ teaspoon cumin

How To:

1. Take a skillet and add olive oil, let it warm over medium-low heat.
2. Add onions, garbanzo and cook for 5 minutes.
3. Stir in spinach, cumin, garbanzo beans and season with sunflower seeds.
4. Use a spoon to smash gently.
5. Cook thoroughly until heated, enjoy!

Nutrition (Per Serving)

- Calories: 90
- Fat: 4g
- Carbohydrates:11g
- Protein:4g

Delicious Garlic Tomatoes

Serving: 4
Prep Time: 10 minutes
Cook Time: 50 minutes
Ingredients:

- 4 garlic cloves, crushed
- 1 pound mixed cherry tomatoes
- 3 thyme sprigs, chopped
- Pinch of sunflower seeds
- Black pepper as needed
- ¼ cup olive oil

How To:

1. Preheat your oven to 325 degrees F.
2. Take a baking dish and add tomatoes, olive oil and thyme.
3. Season with sunflower seeds and pepper and mix.
4. Bake for 50 minutes.
5. Divide tomatoes and pan juices and serve.
6. Enjoy!

Nutrition (Per Serving)

- Calories: 100
- Fat: 0g
- Carbohydrates: 1g
- Protein: 6g

Mashed Celeriac

Serving: 4
Prep Time: 10 minutes
Cook Time: 20 minutes
Ingredients:

- 2 celeriac, washed, peeled and diced
- 2 teaspoons extra-virgin olive oil
- 1 tablespoon honey
- ½ teaspoon ground nutmeg
- Sunflower seeds and pepper as needed

How To:

1. Pre-heat your oven to 400 degrees F.
2. Line a baking sheet with aluminum foil and keep it on the side.
3. Take a large bowl and toss celeriac and olive oil.
4. Spread celeriac evenly on a baking sheet.
5. Roast for 20 minutes until tender.
6. Transfer to a large bowl.
7. Add honey and nutmeg.
8. Use a potato masher to mash the mixture until fluffy.
9. Season with sunflower seeds and pepper.
10. Serve and enjoy!

Nutrition (Per Serving)

- Calories: 136
- Fat: 3g
- Carbohydrates: 26g
- Protein: 4g

Spicy Wasabi Mayonnaise

Serving: 4
Prep Time: 15 minutes
Cook Time: Nil
Ingredients:

- 1 cup mayonnaise
- ½ tablespoon wasabi paste

How To:
1. Take a bowl and mix wasabi paste and mayonnaise.
2. Mix well.
3. Let it chill and use as needed.

Nutrition (Per Serving)

- Calories: 388
- Fat: 42g
- Carbohydrates: 1g
- Protein: 1g

Mediterranean Kale Dish

Serving: 6
Prep Time: 15 minutes
Cook Time: 10 minutes
Ingredients:

- 12 cups kale, chopped
- 2 tablespoons lemon juice
- 1 tablespoon olive oil
- 1 teaspoon coconut aminos
- Sunflower seeds and pepper as needed

How To:
1. Add a steamer insert to your saucepan.
2. Fill the saucepan with water up to the bottom of the steamer.
3. Cover and bring water to boil (medium-high heat).
4. Add kale to the insert and steam for 7-8 minutes.
5. Take a large bowl and add lemon juice, olive oil, sunflower seeds, coconut aminos, and pepper.
6. Mix well and add the steamed kale to the bowl.
7. Toss and serve.
8. Enjoy!

Nutrition (Per Serving)

- Calories: 350
- Fat: 17g
- Carbohydrates: 41g
- Protein: 11g

Spicy Kale Chips

Serving: 4
Prep Time: 10 minutes
Cook Time: 25 minutes
Ingredients:

- 3 cups kale, stemmed and thoroughly washed, torn in 2-inch pieces
- 1 tablespoon extra-virgin olive oil
- ½ teaspoon chili powder
- ¼ teaspoon sea sunflower seeds

How To:

1. Pre-heat your oven to 300 degrees F.
2. Line 2 baking sheets with parchment paper and keep it on the side.
3. Dry kale entirely and transfer to a large bowl.
4. Add olive oil and toss.
5. Make sure each leaf is covered.
6. Season kale with chili powder and sunflower seeds, toss again.
7. Divide kale between baking sheets and spread into a single layer.
8. Bake for 25 minutes until crispy.
9. Cool the chips for 5 minutes and serve.
10. Enjoy!

Nutrition (Per Serving)

- Calories: 56
- Fat: 4g
- Carbohydrates: 5g
- Protein: 2g

Seemingly Easy Portobello Mushrooms

Serving: 4
Prep Time: 10 minutes
Cook Time: 10 minutes
Ingredients:

- 12 cherry tomatoes
- 2 ounces scallions
- 4 portabella mushrooms
- 4 ¼ ounces almond butter
- Sunflower seeds and pepper to taste

How To:

1. Take a large skillet and melt almond butter over medium heat.
2. Add mushrooms and sauté for 3 minutes.
3. Stir in cherry tomatoes and scallions.
4. Sauté for 5 minutes.
5. Season accordingly.
6. Sauté until veggies are tender.
7. Enjoy!

Nutrition (Per Serving)

- Calories: 154
- Fat: 10g
- Carbohydrates: 2g
- Protein: 7g

The Garbanzo Bean Extravaganza

Serving: 5
Prep Time: 10 minutes
Cook Time: Nil
Smart Points: 5
Ingredients:

- 1 can garbanzo beans, chickpeas
- 1 tablespoon olive oil
- 1 teaspoon sunflower seeds
- 1 teaspoon garlic powder
- ½ teaspoon paprika

How To:

1. Pre-heat your oven to 375 degrees F.
2. Line a baking sheet with a silicone baking mat.
3. Drain and rinse garbanzo beans, pat garbanzo beans dry and put into a large bowl.
4. Toss with olive oil, sunflower seeds, garlic powder, paprika and mix well.
5. Spread over a baking sheet.
6. Bake for 20 minutes.
7. Turn chickpeas so they are roasted well.
8. Place back in oven and bake for another 25 minutes at 375 degrees F.
9. Let them cool and enjoy!

Nutrition (Per Serving)

- Calories: 395
- Fat: 7g
- Carbohydrates: 52g
- Protein: 35g

Classic Guacamole

Serving: 6
Prep Time: 15 minutes
Cook Time: Nil
Ingredients:

- 3 large ripe avocados
- 1 large red onion, peeled and diced
- 4 tablespoons freshly squeezed lime juice
- Sunflower seeds as needed
- Freshly ground black pepper as needed
- Cayenne pepper as needed

How To:

1. Halve the avocados and discard stone.
2. Scoop flesh from 3 avocado halves and transfer to a large bowl.
3. Mash using a fork.
4. Add 2 tablespoons of lime juice and mix.
5. Dice the remaining avocado flesh (remaining half) and transfer to another bowl.
6. Add remaining juice and toss.
7. Add diced flesh with the mashed flesh and mix.
8. Add chopped onions and toss.
9. Season with sunflower seeds, pepper and cayenne pepper.
10. Serve and enjoy!

Nutrition (Per Serving)

- Calories: 172
- Fat: 15g
- Carbohydrates: 11g
- Protein: 2g

Apple Slices

Serving: 4
Prep Time: 10 minutes
Cook Time: 10 minutes
Smart Points: 1
Ingredients:

- 1 cup of coconut oil
- ¼ cup date paste
- 2 tablespoons ground cinnamon
- 4 granny smith apples, peeled and sliced, cored

How To:

1. Take a large sized skillet and place it over medium heat.
2. Add oil and allow the oil to heat up.
3. Stir in cinnamon and date paste into the oil.
4. Add cut up apples and cook for 5-8 minutes until crispy.
5. Serve and enjoy!

Nutrition (Per Serving)

- Calories: 368
- Fat: 23g
- Carbohydrates: 44g
- Protein: 1g

Elegant Cashew Sauce

Serving: 4
Prep Time: 5 minutes
Cook Time: Nil
Ingredients:

- 3 ounces cashew nuts
- ¼ cup water
- ½ cup olive oil
- 1 tablespoons lemon juice
- ½ teaspoon onion powder
- ½ teaspoon sunflower seeds
- 1 pinch cayenne pepper

How To:

1. Add nuts to your blender and process.
2. Add other ingredients (except oil) and process until smooth .
3. Add a little bit of oil and puree .
4. Serve as needed!

Nutrition (Per Serving)

- Calories: 361
- Fat: 37g
- Carbohydrates: 6g
- Protein: 3g

Lovely Japanese Cabbage Dish

Serving: 6
Prep Time: 25 minute
Cook Time: Nil
Ingredients:

- 3 tablespoons sesame oil
- 3 tablespoons rice vinegar
- 1 garlic clove, minced
- 1 teaspoon fresh ginger root, grated
- 1 teaspoon sunflower seeds
- 1 teaspoon pepper
- ½ large head cabbage, cored and shredded
- 1 bunch green onions, thinly sliced
- 1 cup almond slivers
- ¼ cup toasted sesame seeds

How To:

1. Add all listed ingredients to a large bowl, making sure to add the wet ingredients first, followed by the dried ingredients.
2. Toss well to ensure that the cabbages are coated well.
3. Let it chill and enjoy!

Nutrition (Per Serving)

- Calories: 126
- Fat: 10g
- Carbohydrates: 9g
- Protein: 4g

Almond Buttery Green Cabbage

Serving: 4
Prep Time: 10 minutes
Cook Time: 15 minutes
Ingredients:

- 1 ½ pounds shredded green cabbage
- 3 ounces almond butter
- Sunflower seeds and pepper to taste
- 1 dollop, whipped cream

How To:

1. Take a large skillet and place it over medium heat.
2. Add almond butter and melt.
3. Stir in cabbage and sauté for 15 minutes.
4. Season accordingly.
5. Serve with a dollop of cream.
6. Enjoy!

Nutrition (Per Serving)

- Calories: 199
- Fat: 17g
- Carbohydrates: 10g
- Protein: 3g

Mesmerizing Brussels and Pistachios

Serving: 4
Prep Time: 15 minutes
Cook Time: 15 minutes
Ingredients:

- 1 pound Brussels sprouts, tough bottom trimmed and halved lengthwise
- 1 tablespoon extra-virgin olive oil
- Sunflower seeds and pepper as needed
- ½ cup roasted pistachios, chopped
- Juice of ½ lemon

How To:

1. Pre-heat your oven to 400 degrees F.
2. Line a baking sheet with aluminum foil and keep it on the side.
3. Take a large bowl and add Brussels sprouts with olive oil and coat well.
4. Season sea sunflower seeds, pepper, spread veggies evenly on sheet.
5. Bake for 15 minutes until lightly caramelized.
6. Remove from oven and transfer to a serving bowl.
7. Toss with pistachios and lemon juice.
8. Serve warm and enjoy!

Nutrition (Per Serving)

- Calories: 126
- Fat: 7g
- Carbohydrates: 14g
- Protein: 6g

Brussels's Fever

Serving: 4
Prep Time: 10 minutes
Cook Time: 20 minutes
Ingredients:

- 2 tablespoons olive oil
- 1 yellow onion, chopped
- 2 pounds Brussels sprouts, trimmed and halved
- 4 cups vegetable stock
- ¼ cup coconut cream

How To:

1. Take a pot and place it over medium heat.
2. Add oil and let it heat up.
3. Add onion and stir-cook for 3 minutes.
4. Add Brussels sprouts and stir, cook for 2 minutes.
5. Add stock and black pepper, stir and bring to a simmer.
6. Cook for 20 minutes more.
7. Use an immersion blender to make the soup creamy.
8. Add coconut cream and stir well.
9. Ladle into soup bowls and serve.
10. Enjoy!

Nutrition (Per Serving)

- Calories: 200
- Fat: 11g
- Carbohydrates: 6g
- Protein: 11g

Hearty Garlic and Kale Platter

Serving: 4
Prep Time: 5 minutes
Cook Time: 10 minutes
Ingredients:

- 1 bunch kale
- 2 tablespoons olive oil
- 4 garlic cloves, minced

How To:

1. Carefully tear the kale into bite sized portions, making sure to remove the stem.
2. Discard the stems.
3. Take a large sized pot and place it over medium heat.
4. Add olive oil and let the oil heat up.
5. Add garlic and stir for 2 minutes.
6. Add kale and cook for 5-10 minutes.
7. Serve!

Nutrition (Per Serving)

- Calories: 121
- Fat: 8g
- Carbohydrates: 5g
- Protein: 4g

Acorn Squash with Mango Chutney

Serving: 4
Prep Time: 10 minutes
Cook Time: 3 hours 10 minutes
Ingredients:

- 1 large acorn squash
- ¼ cup mango chutney
- ¼ cup flaked coconut
- Salt and pepper as needed

How To:

1. Cut the squash into quarters and remove the seeds, discard the pulp.
2. Spray your cooker with olive oil.
3. Transfer the squash to the Slow Cooker and place lid.
4. Take a bowl and add coconut and chutney, mix well and divide the mixture into the center of the Squash.
5. Season well.
6. Place lid on top and cook on LOW for 2-3 hours.
7. Enjoy !

Nutrition (Per Serving)

- Calories: 226
- Fat: 6g
- Carbohydrates: 24g
- Protein: 17g

Satisfying Honey and Coconut Porridge

Serving: 8
Prep Time: 10 minutes
Cook Time: 8 hours
Ingredients:

- 4 cups light coconut milk
- 3 cups apple juice
- 2 ¼ cups coconut flour
- 1 teaspoon ground cinnamon
- ¼ cup honey

How To:

1. In a Slow Cooker, add the coconut milk, apple juice, flour, cinnamon and honey.
2. Stir well.
3. Close lid and cook on LOW for 8 hours.
4. Open lid and stir.
5. Serve with an additional seasoning of fresh fruits.
6. Enjoy!

Nutrition (Per Serving)

- Calories: 372
- Fat: 14g
- Carbohydrates: 56g
- Protein: 8g

Pure Maple Glazed Carrots

Serving: 6
Prep Time: 10 minutes
Cook Time: 8 hours
Ingredients:

- ¼ cup pure maple syrup
- ½ teaspoon ground ginger
- ¼ teaspoon ground nutmeg
- ½ teaspoon salt
- Juice of 1 orange
- 1 pound baby carrots

How To:

1. Take a small bowl and whisk in syrup, nutmeg, ginger, salt, orange juice.
2. Add carrots to your Slow Cooker and pour the maple syrup.
3. Toss to coat.
4. Close lid and cook on LOW for 8 hours.
5. Serve and enjoy!

Nutrition (Per Serving)

- Calories: 76
- Fat: 1g
- Carbohydrates: 19g
- Protein: 76g

Ginger and Orange "Beets"

Serving: 6
Prep Time: 20 minutes
Cook Time: 8 hours
Ingredients:

- 2 pounds beets, peeled and cut into wedges
- Juice of 2 oranges
- Zest of 1 orange
- 1 teaspoon fresh ginger, grated
- 1 tablespoon honey
- 1 tablespoon apple cider vinegar
- 1/8 teaspoon fresh ground black pepper
- Sea salt

How To:

1. Add beets, zest, orange juice, ginger, honey, pepper, salt and vinegar to your Slow Cooker.
2. Stir well.
3. Close lid and cook on LOW for 8 hours.
4. Serve and enjoy!

Nutrition (Per Serving)

- Calories: 108
- Fat: 1g
- Carbohydrates: 25g
- Protein: 3g

Pineapple Rice

Serving: 2
Prep Time: 10 minutes
Cook Time: 2 hours
Ingredients:

- 1 cup rice
- 2 cups water
- 1 small cauliflower, florets separated and chopped
- ½ small pineapple, peeled and chopped
- Salt and pepper as needed
- 1 teaspoon olive oil

How To:

1. Add rice, cauliflower, pineapple, water, oil, salt and pepper to your Slow Cooker.
2. Gently stir.
3. Place lid and cook on HIGH for 2 hours.
4. Fluff the rice with fork and season with more salt and pepper if needed.
5. Divide between serving platters and enjoy!

Nutrition (Per Serving)

- Calories: 152
- Fat: 4g
- Carbohydrates: 18g
- Protein: 4g

Creative Lemon and Broccoli Dish

Serving: 6
Prep Time: 10 minutes
Cook Time: 15 minutes
Ingredients:

- 2 heads broccocli, separated into florets
- 2 teaspoons extra virgin olive oil
- 1 teaspoon sunflower seeds
- ½ teaspoon black pepper
- 1 garlic clove, minced
- ½ teaspoon lemon juice

How To:

1. Pre-heat your oven to 400 degrees F.
2. Take a large sized bowl and add broccoli florets.
3. Drizzle olive oil and season with pepper, sunflower seeds and garlic.
4. Spread broccoli out in a single even layer on a baking sheet.
5. Bake for 15-20 minutes until fork tender.
6. Squeeze lemon juice on top.
7. Serve and enjoy!

Nutrition (Per Serving)

- Calories: 49
- Fat: 1.9g
- Carbohydrates: 7g
- Protein: 3g

Baby Potatoes

Serving: 4
Prep Time: 10 minutes
Cook Time: 35 minutes
Ingredients:

- 2 pounds new yellow potatoes, scrubbed and cut into wedges
- 2 tablespoons extra virgin olive oil
- 2 teaspoons fresh rosemary, chopped
- 1 teaspoon garlic powder
- ½ teaspoon freshly ground black pepper and sunflower seeds

How To:

1. Pre-heat your oven to 400 degrees F.
2. Line a baking sheet with aluminum foil and set it aside.
3. Take a large bowl and add potatoes, olive oil, garlic, rosemary, sea sunflower seeds and pepper.
4. Spread potatoes in a single layer on a baking sheet and bake for 35 minutes.
5. Serve and enjoy!

Nutrition (Per Serving)

- Calories: 225
- Fat: 7g
- Carbohydrates: 37g
- Protein: 5g

Cauliflower Cakes

Serving: 4
Prep Time: 10 minutes
Cook Time: 10 minutes
Ingredients:

- 4 cups cauliflowers, cut into florets
- 1 cup kite ricotta/cashew cheese, grated
- 2 eggs, lightly beaten
- 1 teaspoon paprika
- 1 teaspoon chili powder
- Sunflower seeds and pepper to taste
- ½ cup fresh parsley, chopped
- 1 tablespoon olive oil

How To:

1. Add cauliflower, cheese, paprika, eggs, chili, sunflower seeds, pepper and parsley into a large sized bowl.
2. Mix well.
3. Drizzle olive oil into frying pan and place over medium-high heat.
4. Shape cauliflower mixture into 12 even patties.
5. Once oil is hot, fry cakes until both sides are golden brown.
6. Serve hot and enjoy!

Nutrition (Per Serving)

- Calories: 180
- Fat: 8g
- Carbohydrates: 6g
- Protein: 8g

Tender Coconut and Cauliflower Rice with Chili

Serving: 4
Prep Time: 20 minutes
Cook Time: 20 minutes
Ingredients:

- 3 cups cauliflower, riced
- 2/3 cups full-fat coconut almond milk
- 1-2 teaspoons sriracha paste
- ¼- ½ teaspoon onion powder
- Sunflower seeds as needed
- Fresh basil for garnish

How To:

1. Take a pan and place it over medium low heat.
2. Add all of the ingredients and stir them until fully combined.
3. Cook for about 5-10 minutes, making sure that the lid is on.
4. Remove the lid and keep cooking until any excess liquid is absorbed.
5. Once the rice is soft and creamy, enjoy!

Nutrition (Per Serving)

- Calories: 95
- Fat: 7g
- Carbohydrates: 4g
- Protein: 1g

Apple Slices

Serving: 4
Prep Time: 10 minutes
Cook Time: 10 minutes
Smart Points: 1
Ingredients:

- 1 cup of coconut oil
- ¼ cup date paste
- 2 tablespoons ground cinnamon
- 4 Granny Smith apples, peeled and sliced, cored

How To:

1. Take a large sized skillet and place it over medium heat.
2. Add oil and allow the oil to heat up.
3. Stir cinnamon and date paste into the oil.
4. Add sliced apples and cook for 5-8 minutes until crispy.
5. Serve and enjoy!

Nutrition (Per Serving)

- Calories: 368
- Fat: 23g
- Carbohydrates: 44g
- Protein: 1g

The Exquisite Spaghetti Squash

Serving: 6
Prep Time: 5 minutes
Cooking Time: 7-8 hours
Ingredients:

- 1 spaghetti squash
- 2 cups water

How To:

1. Wash squash carefully with water and rinse it well.
2. Puncture 5-6 holes in the squash using a fork.
3. Place squash in Slow Cooker.
4. Place lid and cook on LOW for 7-8 hours.
5. Remove squash to cutting board and let it cool.
6. Cut squash in half and discard seeds.
7. Use two forks and scrape out squash strands and transfer to bowl.
8. Serve and enjoy!

Nutrition (Per Serving)

- Calories: 52
- Fat: 0g
- Carbohydrates: 12g
- Protein: 1g

The Hearty Garlic and Mushroom Crunch

Serving: 6
Prep Time: 10 minutes
Cooking Time: 8 hours
Ingredients:

- ¼ cup vegetable stock
- 2 tablespoons extra virgin olive oil
- 1 tablespoon Dijon mustard
- 1 teaspoon dried thyme
- 1 teaspoon sea salt
- ½ teaspoon dried rosemary
- ¼ teaspoon fresh ground black pepper
- 2 pounds cremini mushrooms, cleaned
- 6 garlic cloves, minced
- ¼ cup fresh parsley, chopped

How To:

1. Take a small bowl and whisk in vegetable stock, mustard, olive oil, salt, thyme, pepper and rosemary.
2. Add mushrooms, garlic and stock mix to your Slow Cooker.
3. Close lid and cook on LOW for 8 hours.
4. Open lid and stir in parsley.
5. Serve and enjoy!

Nutrition (Per Serving)

- Calories: 92
- Fat: 5g
- Carbohydrates: 8g
- Protein: 4g

Easy Pepper Jack Cauliflower

Serving: 6
Prep Time: 10 minutes
Cooking Time: 3 hours 35 minutes
Ingredients:

- 1 head cauliflower
- ¼ cup whipping cream
- 4 ounces cream cheese
- ½ teaspoon pepper
- 1 teaspoon salt
- 2 tablespoons butter
- 4 ounces pepper jack cheese

How To:

1. Grease slow cooker and add listed ingredients.
2. Stir and place lid, cook on LOW for 3 hours.
3. Remove lid and add cheese, stir.
4. Place lid and cook for 1 hour more.
5. Enjoy!

Nutrition (Per Serving)

- Calories: 272
- Fat: 21g
- Carbohydrates: 5g
- Protein: 10g

The Brussels Platter

Serving: 4
Prep Time: 15 minutes
Cooking Time: 4 hours
Ingredients:

- 1 pound Brussels sprouts, bottoms trimmed and cut
- 1 tablespoon olive oil
- 1 ½ tablespoons Dijon mustard
- Salt and pepper to taste
- ½ teaspoon dried tarragon

How To:

1. Add Brussels sprouts, mustard, water, salt and pepper to your Slow Cooker
2. Add dried tarragon.
3. Stir well and cover.
4. Cook on LOW for 5 hours, making sure to keep cooking until the Brussels sprouts are tender.
5. Stir well and arrange.
6. Add Dijon over the Brussels sprouts.
7. Enjoy!

Nutrition (Per Serving)

- Calories: 83
- Fat: 4g
- Carbohydrates: 11g
- Protein: 4g

The Crazy Southern Salad

Serving: 2
Prep Time: 10 minutes
Cook Time: nil
Ingredients:

- 5 cups Romaine lettuce
- ½ cup sprouted black beans
- 1 cup cherry tomatoes, halved
- 1 avocado, diced
- ¼ cup almonds, chopped
- ½ cup of fresh cilantro
- ½ cup of Salsa Fresca

How To:

1. Take a large sized bowl and add lettuce, tomatoes, beans, almonds, cilantro, avocado, Salsa Fresco
2. Toss everything well and mix them
3. Divide the salad into serving bowls and serve!
4. Enjoy!

Nutrition (Per Serving)

- Calories: 211
- Fat: 16g
- Carbohydrates: 6g
- Protein: 10g

Kale and Carrot with Tahini Dressing

Serving: 1
Prep Time: 15 minutes
Cook Time: nil
Ingredients:

- Handful of kale
- 1 tablespoon tahnini
- ½ head lettuce
- Pinch of garlic powder
- 1 tablespoon olive oil
- Juice of ½ lime
- 1 carrot, grated

How To:

1. Add kale and roughly chopped lettuce to a bowl.
2. Add grated carrots to the greens and mix.
3. Take a small bowl and add the remaining ingredients, mix well.
4. Pour dressing on top of greens and toss.
5. Enjoy!

Nutrition (Per Serving)

- Calories: 249
- Fat: 11g
- Carbohydrates: 35g
- Protein: 10g

Crispy Kale

Serving: 4
Prep Time: 10 minutes
Cook Time: 25 minutes
Ingredients:

- 3 cups kale, stemmed and thoroughly washed, torn in 2-inch pieces
- 1 tablespoon extra-virgin olive oil
- ½ teaspoon chili powder
- ¼ teaspoon sea salt

How To:

1. Prepare your oven by pre-heating to 300 degrees F.
2. Line 2 baking sheets with parchment paper and keep them on the side.
3. Dry kale and transfer to a large bowl.
4. Add olive oil and toss, making sure to cover the leaves well.
5. Season kale with salt, chili powder and toss.
6. Divide kale between baking sheets and spread into single layer.
7. Bake for 25 minutes until crispy.
8. Let them cool for 5 minutes, serve.
9. Enjoy!

Nutrition (Per Serving)

- Calories: 56
- Fat: 4g
- Carbohydrates: 5g
- Protein: 2g

Juicy Summertime Veggies

Serving: 6
Prep Time: 10 minutes
Cooking Time: 3 hours 5 minutes
Ingredients:

- 1 cup grape tomatoes
- 2 cups okra
- 1 cup mushrooms
- 2 cups yellow bell peppers
- 1 ½ cup red onions
- 2 ½ cups zucchini
- ½ cup olive oil
- ½ cup balsamic vinegar
- 1 tablespoon fresh thyme, chopped
- 2 tablespoons fresh basil, chopped

How To:

1. Slice and chop okra, onions, tomatoes, zucchini, mushrooms.
2. Add veggies to a large container and mix.
3. Take another dish and add oil and vinegar, mix in thyme and basil.
4. Toss the veggies into the Slow Cooker and pour marinade.
5. Stir well.
6. Close lid and cook on 3 hours on HIGH, making sure to stir after every hour.

Nutrition (Per Serving)

- Calories: 233
- Fat: 18g
- Carbohydrates: 14g
- Protein: 3g

Crazy Caramelized Onion

Serving: 4
Prep Time: 10 minutes
Cooking Time: 9-10 hours
Ingredients:

- 6 onions, sliced
- 2 tablespoons oil
- ½ teaspoon salt

How To:

1. Add onions, oil and salt to your Slow Cooker.
2. Close lid and cook on LOW for 8 hours.
3. Open lid and keep simmering for 1-2 hours until any excess water has evaporated.
4. Serve and enjoy!

Nutrition (Per Serving)

- Calories: 126
- Fat: 15g
- Carbohydrates: 15g
- Protein: 2g

Kidney Beans and Cilantro

Serving: 6
Prep Time: 5 minutes
Cook Time: nil
Ingredients:

- 1 can (15 ounces) kidney beans, drained and rinsed
- ½ English cucumber, chopped
- 1 medium heirloom tomato, chopped
- 1 bunch fresh cilantro, stems removed and chopped
- 1 red onion, chopped
- Juice of 1 large lime
- 3 tablespoons Dijon mustard
- ½ teaspoon fresh garlic paste
- 1 teaspoon Sumac
- Salt and pepper as needed

How To:

1. Take a medium-sized bowl and add kidney beans, chopped up veggies and cilantro.
2. Take a small bowl and make the vinaigrette by adding lime juice, oil, fresh garlic, pepper, mustard and Sumac.
3. Pour the vinaigrette over the salad and give it a gentle stir.
4. Add some salt and pepper.
5. Cover and allow to chill for half an hour.
6. Serve!

Nutrition (Per Serving)

- Calories: 74
- Fat: 0.7g
- Carbohydrates: 16g
- Protein: 21g

Broccoli Crunchies

Serving: 4
Prep Time: 10 minutes
Cooking Time: 3 hours
Ingredients:

- 2 cups broccoli florets
- 2 ounces cream of celery soup
- 2 tablespoons cheddar cheese, shredded
- 1 small yellow onion, chopped
- ¼ teaspoon Worcestershire sauce
- Salt and pepper as needed
- ½ tablespoon butter

How To:

1. Add broccoli, cream, cheese, onion, cheddar to Slow Cooker.
2. Stir and season with salt and pepper.
3. Place lid and cook on LOW for 3 hours.
4. Serve and enjoy!

Nutrition (Per Serving)

- Calories: 162
- Fat: 11g
- Carbohydrates: 11g
- Protein: 5g

Ultimate Buffalo Cashews

Serving: 4
Prep Time: 10 minutes
Cook Time: 55 minutes
Ingredients:

- 2 cups raw cashews
- ¾ cup red hot sauce
- 1/3 cup avocado oil
- ½ teaspoon garlic powder
- ¼ teaspoon turmeric

How To:

1. Take a bowl, mix the wet ingredients in a bowl and stir in seasoning.
2. Add cashews to the bowl and mix.
3. Soak cashews in hot sauce mix for 2-4 hours.
4. Pre-heat your oven to 325 degrees F.
5. Spread cashews onto baking sheet.
6. Bake for 35-55 minutes, turning after every 10-15 minutes.
7. Let them cool and serve!

Nutrition (Per Serving)

- Calories: 268
- Fat: 16g
- Carbohydrates: 20g
- Protein: 14g

A Green Bean Mixture

Serving: 2
Prep Time: 10 minutes
Cooking Time: 2 hours
Ingredients:

- 4 cups green beans, trimmed
- 2 tablespoons butter, melted
- 1 tablespoon date paste
- Salt and pepper as needed
- ¼ teaspoon coconut aminos

How To:

1. 1. Add green beans, date paste, pepper, salt, coconut aminos to the Slow Cooker, gently stir.
2. Toss and place lid.
3. Cook on LOW for 2 hours.
4. Serve and enjoy!

Nutrition (Per Serving)

- Calories: 236
- Fat: 6g
- Carbohydrates: 10g
- Protein: 6g

Decisive Cauliflower and Mushroom Risotto

Serving: 4
Prep Time: 10 minutes
Cook Time: 20 minutes
Ingredients:

- 1 cup vegetable stock
- 1 head cauliflower, grated
- 9 ounces mushroom, chopped
- 2 tablespoons almond butter
- Sunflower seeds and black pepper, to taste
- 1 cup coconut cream

How To:

1. Take a saucepan and pour stock into it.
2. Bring it to boil and set it aside.
3. Then take a skillet and melt almond butter over medium heat.
4. Add mushroom to sauté until it turns golden brown.
5. Stir in stock and grated cauliflower.
6. Bring the mixture to a simmer and add cream.
7. Cook until liquid is reduced and cauliflower is al dente.
8. Serve warm and enjoy!

Nutrition (Per Serving)

- Calories: 186
- Fat: 16.5g
- Carbohydrates: 6.7g
- Protein: 2.8g

Authentic Zucchini Boats

Serving: 4
Prep Time: 10 minutes
Cook Time: 25 minutes
Smart Points: 3
Ingredients:

- 4 medium zucchini
- ½ cup marinara sauce
- ¼ red onion, sliced
- ¼ cup kalamata olives, chopped
- ½ cup cherry tomatoes, sliced
- 2 tablespoons fresh basil

How To:

1. Pre-heat your oven to 400 degrees F.
2. Cut the zucchini half-lengthwise and shape them in boats.
3. Take a bowl and add tomato sauce, spread 1 layer of sauce on top of each of the boat.
4. Top with onion, olives, and tomatoes.
5. Bake for 20-25 minutes.
6. Top with basil and enjoy!

Nutrition (Per Serving)

- Calories: 278
- Fat: 20g
- Carbohydrates: 10g
- Protein: 15g

Roasted Onions and Green Beans

Serving: 6
Prep Time: 10 minutes
Cook Time: 15 minutes
Ingredients:

- 1 yellow onion, sliced into rings
- ½ teaspoon onion powder
- 2 tablespoons coconut flour
- 1 1/3 pounds fresh green beans, trimmed and chopped

How To:

1. Take a large bowl and mix sunflower seeds with onion powder and coconut flour.
2. Add onion rings.
3. Mix well to coat.
4. Spread the rings in the baking sheet, lined with parchment paper.
5. Drizzle with some oil.
6. Bake for 10 minutes at 400 degrees F.
7. Parboil the green beans for 3 to 5 minutes in the boiling water.
8. Drain and serve the beans with baked onion rings.
9. Serve warm and enjoy!

Nutrition (Per Serving)

- Calories: 214
- Fat: 19.4g
- Carbohydrates:3.7g
- Protein: 8.3g

Chapter 7: Soup Recipes

Hearty Ginger Soup

Serving: 4
Prep Time: 5 minutes
Cook Time: 5 minutes
Ingredients:

- 3 cups coconut almond milk
- 2 cups water
- ½ pound boneless chicken breast halves, cut into chunks
- 3 tablespoons fresh ginger root, minced
- 2 tablespoons fish sauce
- ¼ cup fresh lime juice
- 2 tablespoons green onions, sliced
- 1 tablespoon fresh cilantro, chopped

How To:

1. Take a saucepan and add coconut almond milk and water.
2. Bring the mixture to a boil and add the chicken strips.
3. Reduce the heat to medium and simmer for 3 minutes.
4. Stir in the ginger, lime juice, and fish sauce.
5. Sprinkle a few green onions and cilantro.
6. Serve!

Nutrition (Per Serving)

- Calories: 415
- Fat: 39g
- Carbohydrates: 8g
- Protein: 14g

Tasty Tofu and Mushroom Soup

Serving: 8
Prep Time: 10 minute
Cook Time: 10 minutes
Ingredients:

- 3 cups prepared dashi stock
- ¼ cup shiitake mushrooms, sliced
- 1 tablespoon miso paste
- 1 tablespoon coconut aminos
- 1/8 cup cubed soft tofu
- 1 green onion, diced

How To:

1. Take a saucepan and add stock, bring to a boil.
2. Add mushrooms, cook for 4 minutes.
3. Take a bowl and add coconut aminos, miso paste and mix well.
4. Pour the mixture into stock and let it cook for 6 minutes on simmer.
5. Add diced green onions and enjoy!

Nutrition (Per Serving)

- Calories: 100
- Fat: 4g
- Carbohydrates: 5g
- Protein: 11

Ingenious Eggplant Soup

Serving: 8
Prep Time: 20 minutes
Cook Time: 15 minutes
Ingredients:

- 1 large eggplant, washed and cubed
- 1 tomato, seeded and chopped
- 1 small onion, diced
- 2 tablespoons parsley, chopped
- 2 tablespoons extra virgin olive oil
- 2 tablespoons distilled white vinegar
- ½ cup parmesan cheese, crumbled
- Sunflower seeds as needed

How To:

1. Pre-heat your outdoor grill to medium-high.
2. Pierce the eggplant a few times using a knife/fork.
3. Cook the eggplants on your grill for about 15 minutes until they are charred.
4. Put aside and allow them to cool.
5. Remove the skin from the eggplant and dice the pulp.
6. Transfer the pulp to a mixing bowl and add parsley, onion, tomato, olive oil, feta cheese and vinegar.
7. Mix well and chill for 1 hour.
8. Season with sunflower seeds and enjoy!

Nutrition (Per Serving)

- Calories: 99
- Fat: 7g
- Carbohydrates: 7g
- Protein:3.4g

Loving Cauliflower Soup

Serving: 6
Prep Time: 10 minutes
Cook Time: 10 minutes
Ingredients:

- 4 cups vegetable stock
- 1 pound cauliflower, trimmed and chopped
- 7 ounces Kite ricotta/cashew cheese
- 4 ounces almond butter
- Sunflower seeds and pepper to taste

How To:

1. Take a skillet and place it over medium heat.
2. Add almond butter and melt.
3. Add cauliflower and sauté for 2 minutes.
4. Add stock and bring mix to a boil.
5. Cook until cauliflower is al dente.
6. Stir in cream cheese, sunflower seeds and pepper.
7. Puree the mix using an immersion blender.
8. Serve and enjoy!

Nutrition (Per Serving)

- Calories: 143
- Fat: 16g
- Carbohydrates: 6g
- Protein: 3.4g

Simple Garlic and Lemon Soup

Serving: 3
Prep Time: 10 minutes
Cook Time: nil
Ingredients:

- 1 avocado, pitted and chopped
- 1 cucumber, chopped
- 2 bunches spinach
- 1 ½ cups watermelon, chopped
- 1 bunch cilantro, roughly chopped
- Juice from 2 lemons
- ½ cup coconut aminos
- ½ cup lime juice

How To:

1. Add cucumber, avocado to your blender and pulse well.
2. Add cilantro, spinach and watermelon and blend.
3. Add lemon, lime juice and coconut amino.
4. Pulse a few more times.
5. Transfer to soup bowl and enjoy!

Nutrition (Per Serving)

- Calories: 100
- Fat: 7g
- Carbohydrates: 6g
- Protein: 3g

Healthy Cucumber Soup

Serving: 4
Prep Time: 14 minutes
Cook Time: Nil
Ingredients:

- 2 tablespoons garlic, minced
- 4 cups English cucumbers, peeled and diced
- ½ cup onions, diced
- 1 tablespoon lemon juice
- 1 ½ cups vegetable broth
- ½ teaspoon sunflower seeds
- ¼ teaspoon red pepper flakes
- ¼ cup parsley, diced
- ½ cup Greek yogurt, plain

How To:

1. Add the listed ingredients to a blender and blend to emulsify (keep aside ½ cup of chopped cucumbers).
2. Blend until smooth.
3. Divide the soup amongst 4 servings and top with extra cucumbers.
4. Enjoy chilled!

Nutrition (Per Serving)

- Calories: 371
- Fat: 36g
- Carbohydrates: 8g
- Protein: 4g

Mushroom Cream Soup

Serving: 4
Prep Time: 5 minutes
Cook Time: 30 minutes
Ingredients:

- 1 tablespoon olive oil
- ½ large onion, diced
- 20 ounces mushrooms, sliced
- 6 garlic cloves, minced
- 2 cups vegetable broth
- 1 cup coconut cream
- ¾ teaspoon sunflower seeds
- ¼ teaspoon black pepper
- 1 cup almond milk

How To:

1. Take a large sized pot and place it over medium heat.
2. Add onion and mushrooms to the olive oil and sauté for 10-15 minutes.
3. Make sure to keep stirring it from time to time until browned evenly.
4. Add garlic and sauté for 10 minutes more.
5. Add vegetable broth, coconut cream, almond milk, black pepper and sunflower seeds.
6. Bring it to a boil and lower the temperature to low.
7. Simmer for 15 minutes.
8. Use an immersion blender to puree the mixture.
9. Enjoy!

Nutrition (Per Serving)

- Calories: 200
- Fat: 17g
- Carbohydrates: 5g
- Protein: 4g

Curious Roasted Garlic Soup

Serving: 10
Prep Time: 10 minutes
Cook Time: 60 minutes
Ingredients:

- 1 tablespoon olive oil
- 2 bulbs garlic, peeled
- 3 shallots, chopped
- 1 large head cauliflower, chopped
- 6 cups vegetable broth
- Sunflower seeds and pepper to taste

How To:

1. Pre-heat your oven to 400 degrees F.
2. Slice ¼ inch top of garlic bulb and place it in aluminum foil.
3. Grease with olive oil and roast in oven for 35 minutes.
4. Squeeze flesh out of the roasted garlic.
5. Heat oil in saucepan and add shallots, sauté for 6 minutes.
6. Add garlic and remaining ingredients.
7. Cover pan and reduce heat to low.
8. Let it cook for 15-20 minutes.
9. Use an immersion blender to puree the mixture.
10. Season soup with sunflower seeds and pepper.
11. Serve and enjoy!

Nutrition (Per Serving)

- Calories: 142
- Fat: 8g
- Carbohydrates: 3.4g
- Protein: 4g

Amazing Roasted Carrot Soup

Serving: 4
Prep Time: 10 minutes
Cook Time: 50 minutes
Ingredients:

- 8 large carrots, washed and peeled
- 6 tablespoons olive oil
- 1 quart broth
- Cayenne pepper to taste
- Sunflower seeds and pepper to taste

How To:

1. Pre-heat your oven to 425 degrees F.
2. Take a baking sheet and add carrots, drizzle olive oil and roast for 30-45 minutes.
3. Put roasted carrots into blender and add broth, puree.
4. Pour into saucepan and heat soup.
5. Season with sunflower seeds, pepper and cayenne.
6. Drizzle olive oil.
7. Serve and enjoy!

Nutrition (Per Serving)

- Calories: 222
- Fat: 18g
- Net Carbohydrates: 7g
- Protein: 5g

Simple Pumpkin Soup

Serving: 4
Prep Time: 5 minutes
Cook Time: 6-8 hours
Ingredients:

- 1 small pumpkin, halved, peeled, seeds removed, cubed
- 2 cups chicken broth
- 1 cup coconut milk
- Pepper and thyme to taste

How To:

1. Add all the ingredients to a crockpot.
2. Close the lid.
3. Cook for 6-8 hours on low.
4. Make a smooth puree by using a blender.
5. Garnish with roasted seeds.
6. Serve and enjoy!

Nutrition (Per Serving)

- Calories: 60
- Fat: 2g
- Net Carbohydrates: 10g
- Protein: 3g

Coconut Avocado Soup

Serving: 4
Prep Time: 5 minutes
Cook Time: 5-10 minutes
Ingredients:

- 2 cups vegetable stock
- 2 teaspoons Thai green curry paste
- Pepper as needed
- 1 avocado, chopped
- 1 tablespoon cilantro, chopped
- Lime wedges
- 1 cup coconut milk

How To:

1. Add milk, avocado, curry paste, pepper to blender and blend.
2. Take a pan and place it over medium heat.
3. Add mixture and heat, simmer for 5 minutes.
4. Stir in seasoning, cilantro and simmer for 1 minute.
5. Serve and enjoy!

Nutrition (Per Serving)

- Calories: 250
- Fat: 30g
- Net Carbohydrates: 2g
- Protein: 4g

Coconut Arugula Soup

Serving: 4
Prep Time: 5 minutes
Cook Time: 5-10 minutes
Ingredients:

- Black pepper as needed
- 1 tablespoon olive oil
- 2 tablespoons chives, chopped
- 2 garlic cloves, minced
- 10 ounces baby arugula
- 2 tablespoons tarragon, chopped
- 4 tablespoons coconut milk yogurt
- 6 cups chicken stock
- 2 tablespoons mint, chopped
- 1 onion, chopped
- ½ cup coconut milk

How To:

1. Take a saucepan and place it over medium-high heat, add oil and let it heat up.
2. Add onion and garlic and fry for 5 minutes.
3. Stir in stock and reduce the heat, let it simmer.
4. Stir in tarragon, arugula, mint, parsley and cook for 6 minutes.
5. Mix in seasoning , chives, coconut yogurt and serve.
6. Enjoy!

Nutrition (Per Serving)

- Calories: 180
- Fat: 14g
- Net Carbohydrates: 20g
- Protein: 2g

Awesome Cabbage Soup

Serving: 3
Prep Time: 7 minutes
Cook Time: 25 minutes
Ingredients:

- 3 cups non-fat beef stock
- 2 garlic cloves, minced
- 1 tablespoon tomato paste
- 2 cups cabbage, chopped
- ½ yellow onion
- ½ cup carrot, chopped
- ½ cup green beans
- ½ cup zucchini, chopped
- ½ teaspoon basil
- ½ teaspoon oregano
- Sunflower seeds and pepper as needed

How To:

1. Grease a pot with non-stick cooking spray.
2. Place it over medium heat and allow the oil to heat up.
3. Add onions, carrots, and garlic and sauté for 5 minutes.
4. Add broth, tomato paste, green beans, cabbage, basil, oregano, sunflower seeds, and pepper.
5. Bring the whole mix to a boil and reduce the heat, simmer for 5-10 minutes until all veggies are tender.
6. Add zucchini and simmer for 5 minutes more.
7. Sever hot and enjoy!

Nutrition (Per Serving)

- Calories: 22
- Fat: 0g
- Carbohydrates: 5g
- Protein: 1g

Ginger Zucchini Avocado Soup

Serving: 3
Prep Time: 7 minutes
Cook Time: 25 minutes
Ingredients:

- 1 red bell pepper, chopped
- 1 big avocado
- 1 teaspoon ginger, grated
- Pepper as needed
- 2 tablespoons avocado oil
- 4 scallions, chopped
- 1 tablespoon lemon juice
- 29 ounces vegetable stock
- 1 garlic clove, minced
- 2 zucchini, chopped
- 1 cup water

How To:

1. Take a pan and place over medium heat, add onion and fry for 3 minutes.
2. Stir in ginger, garlic and cook for 1 minute.
3. Mix in seasoning, zucchini stock, water and boil for 10 minutes.
4. Remove soup from fire and let it sit, blend in avocado and blend using an immersion blender.
5. Heat over low heat for a while.
6. Adjust your seasoning and add lemon juice, bell pepper.
7. Serve and enjoy!

Nutrition (Per Serving)

- Calories: 155
- Fat: 11g
- Carbohydrates: 10g
- Protein: 7g

Greek Lemon and Chicken Soup
Serving: 4
Prep Time: 15 minutes
Cook Time: 30 minutes

Ingredients:

- 2 cups cooked chicken, chopped
- 2 medium carrots, chopped
- ½ cup onion, chopped
- ¼ cup lemon juice
- 1 clove garlic, minced
- 1 can cream of chicken soup, fat-free and low sodium
- 2 cans chicken broth, fat-free
- ¼ teaspoon ground black pepper
- 2/3 cup long-grain rice
- 2 tablespoons parsley, snipped

How To:

1. Add all of the listed ingredients to a pot (except rice and parsley).
2. Season with sunflower seeds and pepper.
3. Bring the mix to a boil over medium-high heat.
4. Stir in rice and set heat to medium.
5. Simmer for 20 minutes until rice is tender.
6. Garnish parsley and enjoy!

Nutrition (Per Serving)

- Calories: 582
- Fat: 33g
- Carbohydrates: 35g
- Protein: 32g

Morning Peach

Serving: 4
Prep Time: 10 minutes
Cook Time: 5 minutes
Ingredients:

- 6 small peaches, cored and cut into wedges
- ¼ cup coconut sugar
- 2 tablespoons almond butter
- ¼ teaspoon almond extract

How To:

1. Take a small pan and add peaches, sugar, butter and almond extract.
2. Toss well.
3. Cook over medium-high heat for 5 minutes, divide the mix into bowls and serve.
4. Enjoy!

Nutrition (Per Serving)

- Calories: 198
- Fat: 2g
- Carbohydrates: 11g
- Protein: 8g

Garlic and Pumpkin Soup

Serving: 4
Prep Time: 10 minutes
Cook Time: 5 hours
Ingredients:

- 1 pound pumpkin chunks
- 1 onion, diced
- 2 cups vegetable stock
- 1 2/3 cups coconut cream
- ½ stick almond butter
- 1 teaspoon garlic, crushed
- 1 teaspoon ginger, crushed
- Pepper to taste

How To:

1. Add all the ingredients into your Slow Cooker.
2. Cook for 4-6 hours on high.
3. Puree the soup by using an immersion blender.
4. Serve and enjoy!

Nutrition (Per Serving)

- Calories: 235
- Fat: 21g
- Carbohydrates: 11g
- Protein: 2g

Butternut and Garlic Soup

Serving: 4
Prep Time: 5 minutes
Cook Time: 35 minutes
Ingredients:

- 4 cups butternut squash, cubed
- 4 cups vegetable broth, stock
- ½ cup low fat cream
- 2 garlic cloves, chopped
- Pepper to taste

How To:

1. Add butternut squash, garlic cloves, broth, salt and pepper in a large pot.
2. Place the pot over medium heat and cover with the lid.
3. Bring to boil and then reduce the temperature.
4. Let it simmer for 30-35 minutes.
5. Blend the soup for 1-2 minutes until you get a smooth mixture.
6. Stir the cream through the soup.
7. Serve and enjoy!

Nutrition (Per Serving)

- Calories: 180
- Fat: 14g
- Carbohydrates: 21g
- Protein: 3g

Minty Avocado Soup

Serving: 4
Prep Time: 10 minute + Chill time
Cook Time: nil
Ingredients:

- 1 avocado, ripe
- 1 cup coconut almond milk, chilled
- 2 romaine lettuce leaves
- 20 mint leaves, fresh
- 1 tablespoon lime juice
- Sunflower seeds, to taste

How To:

1. Turn on your slow cooker and add all the ingredients into it.
2. Mix them in a food processor.
3. Make a smooth mixture.
4. Let it chill for 10 minutes.
5. Serve and enjoy!

Nutrition (Per Serving)

- Calories: 280
- Fat: 26g
- Carbohydrates: 12g
- Protein: 4g

Celery, Cucumber and Zucchini Soup

Serving: 2
Prep Time: 10 minute + Chill time
Cook Time: nil
Ingredients:

- 3 celery stalks, chopped
- 7 ounces cucumber, cubed
- 1 tablespoon olive oil
- 2/5 cup fresh cream, 30%, low fat
- 1 red bell pepper, chopped
- 1 tablespoon dill, chopped
- 10 ½ ounces zucchini, cubed
- Sunflower seeds and pepper, to taste

How To:

1. Put the vegetables in a juicer and juice.
2. Then mix in the olive oil and fresh cream.
3. Season with sauce and pepper.
4. Garnish with dill.
5. Serve it chilled and enjoy!

Nutrition (Per Serving)

- Calories: 325
- Fat: 32g
- Carbohydrates: 10g
- Protein: 4g

Rosemary and Thyme Cucumber Soup

Serving: 3
Prep Time: 10 minute + Chill time
Cook Time: nil
Ingredients:

- 4 cups vegetable broth
- 1 teaspoon thyme, freshly chopped
- 1 teaspoon rosemary, freshly chopped
- 2 cucumbers, sliced
- 1 cup low fat cream
- 1 pinch of sunflower seeds

How To:

1. Take a large mixing bowl and add all the ingredients.
2. Whisk well.
3. Blend until smooth by using an immersion blender.
4. Let it chill for 1 hour.
5. Serve and enjoy!

Nutrition (Per Serving)

- Calories: 111
- Fat: 8g
- Carbohydrates: 4g
- Protein: 5g

Guacamole Soup

Serving: 3
Prep Time: 10 minute + Chill time
Cook Time: nil
Ingredients:

- 3 cups vegetable broth
- 2 ripe avocados, pitted
- ½ cup cilantro, freshly chopped
- 1 tomato, chopped
- ½ cup low fat cream
- Sunflower seeds & black pepper, to taste

How To:

1. Add all the ingredients into a blender.
2. Blend until creamy by using an immersion blender.
3. Let it chill for 1 hour.
4. Serve and enjoy!

Nutrition (Per Serving)

- Calories: 289
- Fat: 26g
- Carbohydrates: 5g
- Protein: 10g

Cucumber and Zucchini Soup

Serving: 3
Prep Time: 10 minute + Chill time
Cook Time: nil
Ingredients:

- 2 tablespoons olive oil
- 1 tablespoon fresh dill
- 2/5 cup fresh cream
- 7 ounces cucumber, cubed
- 10 ½ zucchini, cubed
- 1 red pepper, chopped
- 3 celery stalks, chopped
- Sunflower seeds and pepper to taste

How To:

1. Add all the veggies in a juice and make a smooth juice.
2. Mix in the fresh cream and olive oil.
3. Season with pepper and sunflower seeds.
4. Garnish with dill.
5. Serve chilled and enjoy!

Nutrition (Per Serving)

- Calories: 100
- Fat: 8g
- Carbohydrates: 4g
- Protein: 2g

Crockpot Pumpkin Soup

Serving: 3
Prep Time: 10 minute
Cook Time: 6-8 hours
Ingredients:

- 1 small pumpkin, halved, peeled, seeds removed, and pulp cubed
- 2 cups chicken broth
- 1 cup of coconut almond milk
- Sunflower seeds, pepper, thyme, and pepper, to taste

How To:

1. Add all the ingredients to a crockpot.
2. Close the lid.
3. Cook for 6-8 hours on LOW.
4. Make a smooth puree by using a blender.
5. Garnish with roasted seeds.
6. Serve and enjoy!

Nutrition (Per Serving)

- Calories: 60
- Fat: 5g
- Carbohydrates: 4g
- Protein: 4g

Tomato Soup

Serving: 3
Prep Time: 10 minute
Cook Time: 6-8 hours
Ingredients:

- 4 cups water or vegetable broth
- 7 large tomatoes, ripe
- ½ cup macadamia nuts, raw
- 1 medium onion, chopped
- Sunflower seeds and pepper to taste

How To:

1. Take a nonstick skillet and add the onion.
2. Brown the onion for 5 minutes.
3. Add all the ingredients to a crockpot.
4. Cook for 6-8 hours on LOW.
5. Make a smooth puree by using a blender.
6. Serve it warm and enjoy!

Nutrition (Per Serving)

- Calories: 145
- Fat: 12g
- Carbohydrates: 8g
- Protein: 6g

Pumpkin, Coconut and Sage Soup

Serving: 3
Prep Time: 10 minute
Cook Time: 30 minutes
Ingredients:

- 1 cup pumpkin, canned
- 6 cups chicken broth
- 1 cup low fat coconut almond milk
- 1 teaspoon sage, chopped
- 3 garlic cloves, peeled
- Sunflower seeds and pepper to taste

How To:

1. Take a stockpot and add all the ingredients except coconut almond milk into it.
2. Place stockpot over medium heat.
3. Let it bring to a boil.
4. Reduce heat to simmer for 30 minutes.
5. Add the coconut almond milk and stir.
6. Serve bacon and enjoy!

Nutrition (Per Serving)

- Calories: 145
- Fat: 12g
- Carbohydrates: 8g
- Protein: 6g

Sweet Potato and Leek Soup

Serving: 6
Prep Time: 10 minutes
Cook Time: 8 hours
Ingredients:

- 6 cups sweet potatoes, peeled and cubed
- 2 leeks, whites and greens, sliced
- 6 cups vegetable stock
- 1 teaspoon dried thyme
- 1 teaspoon salt
- ¼ teaspoon fresh ground black pepper

How To:

1. Add sweet potatoes, leeks, thyme, stock, salt and pepper to your Slow Cooker.
2. Close lid and cook on LOW for 8 hours.
3. Mash with potato masher/ use an immersion blender to smooth the soup.
4. Serve and enjoy!

Nutrition (Per Serving)

- Calories: 234
- Fat: 2g
- Carbohydrates: 47g
- Protein: 8g

The Kale and Spinach Soup

Serving: 4
Prep Time: 5 minutes
Cook Time: 10 minutes
Ingredients:

- 3 ounces coconut oil
- 8 ounces kale, chopped
- 2 avocado, diced
- 4 1/3 cups coconut almond milk
- Sunflower seeds and pepper to taste

How To:

1. Take a skillet and place it over medium heat.
2. Add kale and sauté for 2-3 minutes
3. Add kale to blender.
4. Add water, spices, coconut almond milk and avocado to blender as well.
5. Blend until smooth and pour mix into bowl.
6. Serve and enjoy!

Nutrition (Per Serving)

- Calories: 124
- Fat: 13g
- Carbohydrates: 7g
- Protein: 4.2g

Japanese Onion Soup

Serving: 4
Prep Time: 15 minutes
Cook Time: 45 minutes
Ingredients:

- ½ stalk celery, diced
- 1 small onion, diced
- ½ carrot, diced
- 1 teaspoon fresh ginger root, grated
- ¼ teaspoon fresh garlic, minced
- 2 tablespoons chicken stock
- 3 teaspoons beef bouillon granules
- 1 cup fresh shiitake, mushrooms
- 2 quarts water
- 1 cup baby Portobello mushrooms, sliced
- 1 tablespoon fresh chives

How To:

1. Take a saucepan and place it over high heat, add water, bring to a boil.
2. Add beef bouillon, celery, onion, chicken stock, carrots, half of the mushrooms, ginger, garlic.
3. Put on the lid and reduce heat to medium, cook for 45 minutes.
4. Take another saucepan and add another half of mushrooms.
5. Once the soup is cooked, strain the soup into the pot with uncooked mushrooms.
6. Garnish with chives and enjoy!

Nutrition (Per Serving)

- Calories: 25
- Fat: 0.2g
- Carbohydrates: 5g
- Protein: 1.4g

Amazing Broccoli and Cauliflower Soup

Serving: 4
Prep Time: 10 minutes
Cooking Time: 8 hours
Ingredients:

- 3 cups broccoli florets
- 2 cups cauliflower florets
- 2 garlic cloves, minced
- ½ cup shallots, chopped
- 1 carrot, chopped
- 3 ½ cups low sodium veggie stick
- Pinch of pepper
- 1 cup fat-free milk
- 6 ounces low-fat cheddar, shredded
- 1 cup non-fat Greek yogurt

How To:

1. Add broccoli, cauliflower, garlic, shallots, carrot, stock, pepper to your Slow Cooker.
2. Stir well and place lid.
3. Cook on LOW for 8 hours.
4. Add milk and cheese.
5. Use an immersion blender to smooth the soup.
6. Add yogurt and blend once more.
7. Ladle into bowls and enjoy!

Nutrition (Per Serving)

- Calories: 218
- Fat: 11g
- Carbohydrates: 15g
- Protein: 12g

Amazing Zucchini Soup

Serving: 4
Prep Time: 10 minutes
Cook Time: 20 minutes
Ingredients:

- 1 onion, chopped
- 3 zucchini, cut into medium chunks
- 2 tablespoons coconut milk
- 2 garlic cloves, minced
- 4 cups chicken stock
- 2 tablespoons coconut oil
- Pinch of salt
- Black pepper to taste

How To:

1. Take a pot and place over medium heat.
2. Add oil and let it heat up.
3. Add zucchini, garlic, onion and stir.
4. Cook for 5 minutes.
5. Add stock, salt, pepper and stir.
6. Bring to a boil and reduce the heat.
7. Simmer for 20 minutes.
8. Remove from heat and add coconut milk.
9. Use an immersion blender until smooth.
10. Ladle into soup bowls and serve.
11. Enjoy!

Nutrition (Per Serving)

- Calories: 160
- Fat: 2g
- Carbohydrates: 4g
- Protein: 7g

Portuguese Kale and Sausage Soup

Serving: 4
Prep Time: 10 minutes
Cook Time: 35 minutes
Ingredients:

- 1 yellow onion, chopped
- 16 ounces sausage, chopped
- 3 sweet potatoes, chopped
- 4 cups chicken stock
- 1 pound kale, chopped
- pepper as needed

How To:
1. Take a pot and place it over medium heat.
2. Add sausage and brown both sides.
3. Transfer to bowl.
4. Heat pot again over medium heat.
5. Add onion and stir for 5 minutes.
6. Add stock, sweet potatoes, stir and bring to a simmer.
7. Cook for 20 minutes.
8. Use an immersion blender to blend.
9. Add kale and pepper and simmer for 2 minutes over low heat.
10. Ladle soup to bowls and top with sausage with pieces.
11. Serve and enjoy!

Nutrition (Per Serving)

- Calories: 200
- Fat: 2g
- Carbohydrates: 6g
- Protein:8g

Dazzling Pizza Soup

Serving: 6
Prep Time: 5 minutes
Cook Time: 30 minutes
Ingredients:

- 12 ounces chicken meat, sliced
- 4 ounces uncured pepperoni
- 1 can 25 ounces marinara
- 1 can 14.5 ounces fire roasted tomatoes
- 1 large onion, diced
- 15 ounces mushrooms, sliced
- 1 can 3 ounce sliced black olives
- 1 tablespoon dried oregano
- 1 teaspoon garlic powder
- ½ teaspoon salt

How To:
1. Take large sized saucepan and add in the peperoni, chicken meat, marinara, onions, tomatoes, mushroom, oregano, olives, salt and garlic powder.
2. Cook the mixture for 30 minutes over medium level heat and soften the mushroom and onions.
3. Serve hot.

Nutrition (Per Serving)

- Calories: 90
- Fat: 2g
- Carbohydrates: 17g
- Protein: 3g

Mesmerizing Lentil Soup

Serving: 4
Prep Time: 10 minutes
Cooking Time: 8 hours
Ingredients:

- 1 pound dried lentils, soaked overnight and rinsed
- 3 carrots, peeled and chopped
- 1 celery stalk, chopped
- 1 onion, chopped
- 6 cups vegetables broth
- 1 ½ teaspoons garlic powder
- 1 teaspoon ground cumin
- 1 teaspoon smoked paprika
- 1 teaspoon dried thyme
- ¼ teaspoon liquid smoke
- ¼ teaspoon salt
- ¼ teaspoon ground pepper

How To:

1. Add listed ingredients to Slow Cooker and stir well.
2. Place lid and cook for 8 hours on LOW.
3. Stir and serve.
4. Enjoy!

Nutrition (Per Serving)

- Calories: 307
- Fat: 1g
- Carbohydrates: 56g
- Protein: 20g

Organically Healthy Chicken Soup

Serving: 4
Prep Time: 10 minutes
Cook Time: 12-15 minutes
Ingredients:

- 2 cans (14 ounces each) low sodium chicken broth
- 2 cups water
- 1 cup twisted spaghetti
- ¼ teaspoon pepper
- 3 cups mixed vegetables (such as broccoli, carrots etc.)
- 1 and ½ cups chicken, cooked and cubed
- 1 tablespoon fresh basil, snipped
- ¼ cup parmesan, finely shredded

How To:

1. Take a Dutch Oven and add broth, water, pepper and bring the mixture to a boil.
2. Gently stir in pasta and wait until the mixture reaches boiling point again,
3. Lower down the heat and let the mixture simmer for 5 minutes (covered).
4. Remove lid and stir in the vegetables, return the mixture boil and lower down heat once again.
5. Cover and let it simmer over low heat for 5-8 minutes until the pasta and veggies and tender and cooked.
6. Stir in cooked chicken and garnish with basil.
7. Serve with a topping of parmesan.
8. Enjoy!

Nutrition Values (Per Serving)

- Calories: 400
- Fat: 9g
- Carbohydrates: 37g
- Protein: 45g

Potato and Asparagus Bisque

Serving: 4
Prep Time: 5 minutes
Cook Time: 6 minutes
Ingredients:

- 1 ½ pound asparagus
- 2 pounds sweet potatoes
- 6 cups vegetable broth
- 1 large sized onion
- 8 cloves garlic
- 2 tablespoons dried dill
- 2 tablespoons flavored vinegar
- 3-4 cups almond milk
- 4 tablespoons Dijon mustard
- 4 tablespoons yeast

How To:

1. Add the listed ingredients (except milk, mustard and yeast) to your pot.
2. Lock the lid and cook on HIGH pressure for 6 minutes.
3. Release the pressure naturally.
4. Open the lid and add almond milk, yeast and mustard.
5. Puree using immersion blender.
6. Serve over rice.
7. Enjoy!

Nutrition (Per Serving)

- Calories: 430
- Fat: 12g
- Carbohydrates: 77g
- Protein: 6g

Cabbage and Leek Soup

Serving: 4
Prep Time: 10 minutes
Cook Time: 25 minutes
Ingredients:

- 2 tablespoons coconut oil
- ½ head chopped up cabbage
- 3-4 diced ribs celery
- 2-3 carefully cleaned and chopped leeks
- 1 diced bell pepper
- 2-3 diced carrots
- 2/3 cloves minced garlic
- 4 cups chicken broth
- 1 teaspoon Italian seasoning
- 1 teaspoon Creole seasoning
- Black pepper as needed
- 2-3 cups mixed salad greens

How To:

1. Set your pot to Sauté mode and add coconut oil.
2. Allow the oil to heat up.
3. Add the veggies (except salad greens) starting from the carrot, making sure to stir well after each vegetable addition.
4. Make sure to add the garlic last.
5. Season with Italian seasoning, black pepper and Creole seasoning.
6. Add broth and lock the lid.

7. Cook on SOUP mode for 20 minutes.
8. Release the pressure naturally and add salad greens, stir well and allow to sit for a while.
9. Allow for a few minutes to wilt the veggies.
10. Season with a bit of flavored vinegar and pepper and enjoy!

Nutrition (Per Serving)

- Calories: 32
- Fat: 0g
- Carbohydrates: 4g
- Protein: 2g

Onion Soup

Serving: 4
Prep Time: 10 minutes
Cook Time: 3 hours
Ingredients:

- 2 tablespoons avocado oil
- 5 yellow onions, cut into halved and sliced
- Black pepper to taste
- 5 cups beef stock
- 3 thyme sprigs
- 1 tablespoon tomato paste

How To:

1. Take a pot and place it over medium high heat.
2. Add onion and thyme and stir.
3. Reduce heat to low and cook for 30 minutes.
4. Uncover pot and cook onions for 1 hour and 30 minutes more, stirring often.
5. Add tomato paste, stock and stir.
6. Simmer for 1 hour more.
7. Ladle soup into bowls and enjoy!

Nutrition (Per Serving)

- Calories: 200
- Fat: 4g
- Carbohydrates: 6g
- Protein: 8g

Carrot, Ginger and Turmeric Soup

Serving: 4
Prep Time: 15 minutes
Cook Time: 40 minutes
Ingredients:

- 6 cups chicken broth
- ¼ cup full fat coconut milk, unsweetened
- ¾ pound carrots, peeled and chopped
- 1 teaspoon turmeric, ground
- 2 teaspoons ginger, grated
- 1 yellow onion, chopped
- 2 garlic cloves, peeled
- Pinch of pepper

How To:

1. Take a stockpot and add all the ingredients except coconut milk into it.
2. Place stockpot over medium heat.
3. Bring to a boil.
4. Reduce heat to simmer for 40 minutes.
5. Remove the bay leaf.
6. Blend the soup until smooth by using an immersion blender.
7. Add the coconut milk and stir.
8. Serve immediately and enjoy!

Nutrition (Per Serving)

- Calories: 79
- Fat: 4g
- Carbohydrates: 7g
- Protein: 4g

Offbeat Squash Soup

Serving: 4
Prep Time: 10 minutes
Cook Time: 50 minutes
Ingredients:

- 1 butternut squash, cut in halve lengthwise and deseeded
- 14 ounces coconut milk
- Pinch of salt
- Black pepper to taste
- Handful of parsley, chopped
- Pinch of nutmeg, ground

How To:

1. Add butternut squash halves on a lined baking sheet.
2. Place in oven and bake for 45 minutes at 350 degrees F.
3. Leave squash to cool down and scoop out the flesh to a pot.
4. Add half of the coconut milk to the pot and blend using immersion blender.
5. Heat soup over medium-low heat and add remaining coconut milk.
6. Add a pinch of salt, black pepper to taste.
7. Add nutmeg, parsley and blend using an immersion blender once again for a few seconds.
8. Cook for 4 minutes.
9. Serve and enjoy!

Nutrition (Per Serving)

- Calories: 144
- Fat: 10g
- Carbohydrates: 7g
- Protein: 2g

Leek and Cauliflower Soup

Serving: 6
Prep Time: 10 minutes
Cook Time: 40 minutes
Ingredients:

- 3 cups cauliflower, riced
- 1 bay leaf
- 1 teaspoon herbs de Provence
- 2 garlic cloves, peeled and diced
- ½ cup coconut milk
- 2 ½ cups vegetable stock
- 1 tablespoon coconut oil
- ½ teaspoon cracked pepper
- 1 leek, chopped

How To:

1. Take a pot, heat oil into it.
2. Sauté the leeks in the oil for 5 minutes.
3. Add the garlic and then stir-cook for another minute.
4. Add all the remaining ingredients and mix them well.
5. Cook for 30 minutes.
6. Stir occasionally.
7. Blend the soup until smooth by using an immersion blender.
8. Serve hot and enjoy!

Nutrition (Per Serving)

- Calories: 90
- Fat: 7g
- Carbohydrates: 4g
- Protein: 2g

Dreamy Zucchini Bowl

Serving: 4
Prep Time: 10 minutes
Cook Time: 20 minutes
Ingredients:

- 1 onion, chopped
- 3 zucchini, cut into medium chunks
- 2 tablespoons coconut almond milk
- 2 garlic cloves, minced
- 4 cups vegetable stock
- 2 tablespoons coconut oil
- Pinch of sunflower seeds
- Black pepper to taste

How To:

1. Take a pot and place it over medium heat.
2. Add oil and let it heat up.
3. Add zucchini, garlic, onion and stir.
4. Cook for 5 minutes.
5. Add stock, sunflower seeds, pepper and stir.
6. Bring to a boil and reduce heat.
7. Simmer for 20 minutes.
8. Remove from heat and add coconut almond milk.
9. Use an immersion blender until smooth.
10. Ladle into soup bowls and serve.
11. Enjoy!

Nutrition (Per Serving)

- Calories: 160
- Fat: 2g
- Carbohydrates: 4g
- Protein: 7g

Cold Crab and Watermelon Soup

Serving: 4
Prep Time: 10 minutes + chill time
Cook Time: nil
Ingredients:

- ¼ cup basil, chopped
- 2 pounds tomatoes
- 5 cups watermelon, cubed
- ¼ cup wine vinegar
- 2 garlic cloves, minced
- 1 zucchini, chopped
- Pepper to taste
- 1 cup crabmeat

How To:

1. Take your blender and add tomatoes, basil, vinegar, 4 cups watermelon, garlic, 1/3 cup oil, pepper and pulse well.
2. Transfer to fridge and chill for 1 hour.
3. Divide into bowls and add zucchini, crab and remaining watermelon.
4. Serve and enjoy!

Nutrition (Per Serving)

- Calories: 121
- Fat: 3g
- Carbohydrates: 4g
- Protein: 8g

Paleo Lemon and Garlic Soup

Serving: 4
Prep Time: 10 minutes
Cook Time: 10 minutes
Ingredients:

- 6 cups shellfish stock
- 1 tablespoon garlic, minced
- 1 tablespoon coconut oil, melted
- 2 whole eggs
- ½ cup lemon juice
- Pinch of salt
- White pepper to taste
- 1 tablespoon arrowroot powder
- Finely chopped cilantro for serving

How To:

1. Heat up a pot with oil over medium high heat.
2. Add garlic, stir cook for 2 minutes.
3. Add stock (reserve ½ cup for later use).
4. Stir and bring mix to a simmer.
5. Take a bowl and add eggs, sea salt, pepper, reserved stock, lemon juice and arrowroot.
6. Whisk well.
7. Pour in to the soup and cook for a few minutes.
8. Ladle soup into bowls and serve with chopped cilantro.
9. Enjoy!

Nutrition (Per Serving)

- Calories: 135
- Fat: 3g
- Carbohydrates: 12g
- Protein: 8

Brussels Soup

Serving: 4
Prep Time: 10 minutes
Cook Time: 20 minutes
Ingredients:

- 2 tablespoons olive oil
- 1 yellow onion, chopped
- 2 pounds Brussels sprouts, trimmed and halved
- 4 cups chicken stock
- ¼ cup coconut cream

How To:

1. Take a pot and place it over medium heat.
2. Add oil and let it heat up.
3. Add onion and stir-cook for 3 minutes.
4. Add Brussels sprouts and stir, cook for 2 minutes.
5. Add stock and black pepper, stir and bring to a simmer.
6. Cook for 20 minutes more.
7. Use an immersion blender to make the soup creamy.
8. Add coconut cream and stir well.
9. Ladle into soup bowls and serve.
10. Enjoy!

Nutrition (Per Serving)

- Calories: 200
- Fat: 11g
- Carbohydrates: 6g
- Protein: 11g

Spring Soup and Poached Egg

Serving: 4
Prep Time: 5 minutes
Cook Time: 15 minutes
Ingredients:

- 2 whole eggs
- 32 ounces chicken broth
- 1 head romaine lettuce, chopped

How To:

1. Bring the chicken broth to a boil.
2. Reduce the heat and poach the 2 eggs in the broth for 5 minutes.
3. Take two bowls and transfer the eggs into a separate bowl.
4. Add chopped romaine lettuce into the broth and cook for a few minutes.
5. Serve the broth with lettuce into the bowls.
6. Enjoy!

Nutrition (Per Serving)

- Calories: 150
- Fat: 5g
- Carbohydrates: 6g
- Protein: 16g

Lobster Bisque

Serving: 4
Prep Time: 10 minutes
Cook Time: 15 minutes
Ingredients:

- ¾ pound lobster, cooked and lobster
- 4 cups chicken broth
- 2 garlic cloves, chopped
- ¼ teaspoon pepper
- ½ teaspoon paprika
- 1 yellow onion, chopped
- ½ teaspoon salt
- 14 ½ ounces tomatoes, diced
- 1 tablespoon coconut oil
- 1 cup low fat cream

How To:

1. Take a stockpot and add the coconut oil over medium heat.
2. Then sauté the garlic and onion for 3 to 5 minutes.
3. Add diced tomatoes, spices and chicken broth and bring to a boil.
4. Reduce to a simmer, then simmer for about 10 minutes.
5. Add the warmed heavy cream to the soup.
6. Blend the soup till creamy by using an immersion blender.
7. Stir in cooked lobster.
8. Serve and enjoy!

Nutrition (Per Serving)

- Calories: 180
- Fat: 11g
- Carbohydrates: 6g
- Protein: 16g

Tomato Bisque

Serving: 4
Prep Time: 10 minutes
Cook Time: 40 minutes
Ingredients:

- 4 cups chicken broth
- 1 cup low fat cream
- 1 teaspoon thyme dried
- 3 cups canned whole, peeled tomatoes
- 2 tablespoons almond butter
- 3 garlic cloves, peeled
- Pepper as needed

How To:

1. Take a stockpot and first add the butter to the bottom of a stockpot.
2. Then add all the ingredients except heavy cream into it.
3. Bring to a boil.
4. Simmer for 40 minutes.
5. Warm the heavy cream and stir into the soup.
6. Serve and enjoy!

Nutrition (Per Serving)

- Calories: 141
- Fat: 12g
- Carbohydrates: 4g
- Protein: 4g

Chipotle Chicken Chowder

Serving: 4
Prep Time: 10 minutes
Cook Time: 23 minutes
Ingredients:

- 1 medium onion, chopped
- 2 garlic cloves, minced
- 6 bacon slices, chopped
- 4 cups jicama, cubed
- 3 cups chicken stock
- 1 teaspoon salt
- 2 cups low-fat, cream
- 1 tablespoon olive oil
- 2 tablespoons fresh cilantro, chopped
- 1 ¼ pounds chicken, thigh boneless, cut into 1 inch chunks
- ½ teaspoon pepper
- 1 chipotle pepper, minced

How To:

1. Heat olive oil over medium heat in a large sized saucepan, add bacon.
2. Cook until crispy, add onion, garlic, and jicama.
3. Cook for 7 minutes, add chicken stock and chicken.
4. Bring to a boil and reduce temperature to low.
5. Simmer for 10 minutes
6. Season with salt and pepper.
7. Add heavy cream and chipotle, simmer for 5 minutes.
8. Sprinkle chopped cilantro and serve, enjoy!

Nutrition (Per Serving)

- Calories: 350
- Fat: 22g
- Carbohydrates: 8g
- Protein: 22g

Bay Scallop Chowder

Serving: 4
Prep Time: 10 minutes
Cook Time: 18 minutes
Ingredients:

- 1 medium onion, chopped
- 2 ½ cups chicken stock
- 4 slices bacon, chopped
- 3 cups daikon radish, chopped
- ½ teaspoon dried thyme
- 2 cups low-fat cream
- 1 tablespoon almond butter
- Pepper to taste
- 1 pound bay scallops

How To:

1. Heat olive over medium heat in a large sized saucepan, add bacon and cook until crisp, add onion and daikon radish.
2. Cook for 5 minutes, add chicken stock.
3. Simmer for 8 minutes, season with salt and pepper, thyme.
4. Add heavy cream, bay scallops, simmer for 4 minutes
5. Serve and enjoy!

Nutrition (Per Serving)

- Calories: 307
- Fat: 22g
- Carbohydrates: 7g
- Protein: 22g

Salmon and Vegetable Soup

Serving: 4
Prep Time: 10 minutes
Cook Time: 22 minutes
Ingredients:

- 2 tablespoons extra-virgin olive oil
- 1 leek, chopped
- 1 red onion, chopped
- Pepper to taste
- 2 carrots, chopped
- 4 cups low stock vegetable stock
- 4 ounces salmon, skinless and boneless, cubed
- ½ cup coconut cream
- 1 tablespoon dill, chopped

How To:

1. Take a pan and place it over medium heat, add leek, onion, stir and cook for 7 minutes.
2. Add pepper, carrots, stock and stir.
3. Boil for 10 minutes.
4. Add salmon, cream, dill and stir.
5. Boil for 5-6 minutes.
6. Ladle into bowls and serve.
7. njoy!

Nutrition (Per Serving)

- Calories: 240
- Fat: 4g
- Carbohydrates: 7g
- Protein: 12g

Garlic Tomato Soup

Serving: 4
Prep Time: 15 minutes
Cook Time: 15 minutes
Ingredients:

- 8 Roma tomatoes, chopped
- 1 cup tomatoes, sundried
- 2 tablespoons coconut oil
- 5 garlic cloves, chopped
- 14 ounces coconut milk
- 1 cup vegetable broth
- Pepper to taste
- Basil, for garnish

How To:

1. Take a pot, heat oil into it.
2. Sauté the garlic in it for ½ minute.
3. Mix in the Roma tomatoes and cook for 8-10 minutes.
4. Stir occasionally.
5. Add in the rest of the ingredients, except the basil, and stir well.
6. Cover the lid and cook for 5 minutes.
7. Let it cool.
8. Blend the soup until smooth by using an immersion blender.
9. Garnish with basil.
10. Serve and enjoy!

Nutrition (Per Serving)

- Calories: 240
- Fat: 23g
- Carbohydrates: 16g
- Protein: 7g

Melon Soup

Serving: 4
Prep Time:6 minutes
Cook Time: Nil
Ingredients:

- 4 cups casaba melon, seeded and cubed
- 1 tablespoon fresh ginger, grated
- ¾ cup coconut milk
- Juice of 2 limes

How To:

1. Add the lime juice, coconut milk, casaba melon, ginger and salt into your blender.
2. Blend for 1-2 minutes until you get a smooth mixture.
3. Serve and enjoy!

Nutrition (Per Serving)

- Calories: 134
- Fat: 9g
- Carbohydrates: 13g
- Protein: 2g

Chapter 8: Seafood Recipes

Spicy Baked Shrimp

Serving: 4
Prep Time: 10 minutes
Cook Time: 25 minutes + 2-4 hours
Ingredients:

- ½ ounce large shrimp, peeled and deveined
- Cooking spray as needed
- 1 teaspoon low sodium coconut aminos
- 1 teaspoon parsley
- ½ teaspoon olive oil
- ½ tablespoon honey
- 1 tablespoon lemon juice

How To:

1. Pre-heat your oven to 450 degrees F.
2. Take a baking dish and grease it well.
3. Mix in all the ingredients and toss.
4. Transfer to oven and bake for 8 minutes until shrimp turns pink.
5. Serve and enjoy!

Nutrition (Per Serving)

- Calories: 321
- Fat: 9g
- Carbohydrates: 44g
- Protein: 22g

Shrimp and Cilantro Meal

Serving: 4
Prep Time: 10 minutes
Cook Time: 5 minutes
SmartPoints: 0
Ingredients:

- 1 ¾ pounds shrimp, deveined and peeled
- 2 tablespoons fresh lime juice
- ¼ teaspoon cloves, minced
- ½ teaspoon ground cumin
- 1 tablespoon olive oil
- 1 ¼ cups fresh cilantro, chopped
- 1 teaspoon lime zest
- ½ teaspoon sunflower seeds
- ¼ teaspoon pepper

Direction

1. Take a large sized bowl and add shrimp, cumin, garlic, lime juice, ginger and toss well.
2. Take a large sized non-stick skillet and add oil, allow the oil to heat up over medium-high heat.
3. Add shrimp mixture and sauté for 4 minutes.
4. Remove the heat and add cilantro, lime zest, sunflower seeds, and pepper.
5. Mix well and serve hot!

Nutrition (Per Serving)

- Calories: 177
- Fat: 6g
- Carbohydrates: 2g
- Protein: 27g

The Original Dijon Fish

Serving: 2
Prep Time: 3 minutes
Cook Time: 12 minutes
SmartPoints: 2
Ingredients:

- 1 perch, flounder or sole fish florets
- 1 tablespoon Dijon mustard
- 1 ½ teaspoons lemon juice
- 1 teaspoon low sodium Worcestershire sauce, low sodium
- 2 tablespoons Italian seasoned bread crumbs
- 1 almond butter flavored cooking spray

How To:

1. Preheat your oven to 450 degrees F.
2. Take an 11 x 7-inch baking dish and arrange your fillets carefully.
3. Take a small sized bowl and add lemon juice, Worcestershire sauce, mustard and mix it well.
4. Pour the mix over your fillet.
5. Sprinkle a good amount of breadcrumbs.
6. Bake for 12 minutes until fish flakes off easily.
7. Cut the fillet in half portions and enjoy!

Nutrition (Per Serving)

- Calories: 125
- Fat: 2g
- Carbohydrates: 6g
- Protein: 21g

Lemony Garlic Shrimp

Serving: 4
Prep Time: 5-10 minutes
Cook Time: 10-15 minutes
Ingredients:

- 1 ¼ pounds shrimp, boiled or steamed
- 3 tablespoons garlic, minced
- ¼ cup lemon juice
- 2 tablespoons olive oil
- ¼ cup parsley

How To:

1. Take a small skillet and place over medium heat, add garlic and oil and stir-cook for 1 minute.
2. Add parsley, lemon juice and season with sunflower seeds and pepper accordingly.
3. Add shrimp in a large bowl and transfer the mixture from the skillet over the shrimp.
4. Chill and serve.
5. Enjoy!

Nutrition (Per Serving)

- Calories: 130
- Fat: 3g
- Carbohydrates:2g
- Protein:22g

Baked Zucchini Wrapped Fish

Serving: 2
Prep Time: 15 minutes
Cook Time: 15 minutes
SmartPoints: 0
Ingredients:

- 24-ounce cod fillets, skin removed
- 1 tablespoon of blackening spices
- 2 zucchini, sliced lengthwise to form ribbon
- ½ tablespoon of olive oil

How To:

1. Season the fish fillets with blackening spice.
2. Wrap each fish fillet with zucchini ribbons.
3. Place fish on a plate.
4. Take a skillet and place over medium heat.
5. Pour oil and allow the oil to heat up.
6. Add wrapped fish to the skillet and cook each side for 4 minutes.
7. Serve and enjoy!

Nutrition (Per Serving)

- Calories: 397
- Fat: 23g
- Carbohydrates: 2g
- Protein: 46g

Heart-Warming Medi Tilapia

Serving: 4
Prep Time: 15 minutes
Cook Time: 15 minute
Ingredients:

- 3 tablespoons sun-dried tomatoes, packed in oil, drained and chopped
- 1 tablespoon capers, drained
- 2 tilapia fillets
- 1 tablespoon oil from sun-dried tomatoes
- 2 tablespoons kalamata olives, chopped and pitted

How To:

1. Pre-heat your oven to 372 degrees F.
2. Take a small sized bowl and add sun-dried tomatoes, olives, capers and stir well.
3. Keep the mixture on the side.
4. Take a baking sheet and transfer the tilapia fillets and arrange them side by side.
5. Drizzle olive oil all over them.
6. Bake in your oven for 10-15 minutes.
7. After 10 minutes, check the fish for a "Flaky" texture.
8. Once cooked, top the fish with the tomato mixture and serve!

Nutrition (Per Serving)

- Calories: 183
- Fat: 8g
-
- Carbohydrates: 18g
- Protein:83g

Baked Salmon and Orange Juice

Serving: 2
Prep Time: 10 minutes
Cook Time: 10 minutes
Ingredients:

- ½ pound salmon steak
- Juice of 1 orange
- Pinch ginger powder, black pepper, and sunflower seeds
- Juice of ½ lemon
- 1-ounce coconut almond milk

How To:

1. Preheat oven to 350 degrees F.
2. Rub salmon steak with spices and let it sit for 15 minutes.
3. Take a bowl and squeeze an orange.
4. Squeeze lemon juice as well and mix.
5. Pour almond milk into the mixture and stir.
6. Take a baking dish and line with aluminum foil.
7. Place steak on it and pour the sauce over steak.
8. Cover with another sheet and bake for 10 minutes.
9. Serve and enjoy!

Nutrition (Per Serving)

- Calories: 300
- Fat: 3g
- Carbohydrates: 1g
- Protein: 7g

Lemon and Almond butter Cod

Serving: 2
Prep Time: 5 minutes
Cook Time: 20 minutes
Ingredients:

- 4 tablespoons almond butter, divided
- 4 thyme sprigs, fresh and divided
- 4 teaspoons lemon juice, fresh and divided
- 4 cod fillets, 6 ounces each
- Sunflower seeds to taste

How To:

1. Pre-heat your oven to 400 degrees F.
2. Season cod fillets with sunflower seeds on both sides.
3. Take four pieces of foil, each foil should be 3 times bigger than the fillets.
4. Divide fillets between the foil and top with almond butter, lemon juice, thyme.
5. Fold to form a pouch and transfer pouches to the baking sheet.
6. Bake for 20 minutes.
7. Open and let the steam out.
8. Serve and enjoy!

Nutrition (Per Serving)

- Calories: 284
- Fat: 18g
- Carbohydrates: 2g
- Protein: 32g

Shrimp Scampi

Serving: 4
Prep Time: 25 minutes
Cook Time: Nil
SmartPoints: 1
Ingredients:

- 4 teaspoons olive oil
- 1 ¼ pounds medium shrimp
- 6-8 garlic cloves, minced
- ½ cup low sodium chicken broth
- ½ cup dry white wine
- ¼ cup fresh lemon juice
- ¼ cup fresh parsley + 1 tablespoon extra, minced
- ¼ teaspoon sunflower seeds
- ¼ teaspoon fresh ground pepper
- 4 slices lemon

How To:

1. Take a large sized bowl and place it over medium-high heat.
2. Add oil and allow the oil to heat up.
3. Add shrimp and cook for 2-3 minutes.
4. Add garlic and cook for 30 seconds.
5. Take a slotted spoon and transfer the cooked shrimp to a serving platter.
6. Add broth, lemon juice, wine, ¼ cup of parsley, pepper, and sunflower seeds to the skillet.
7. Bring the whole mix to a boil.
8. Keep boiling until the sauce has been reduced to half.
9. Spoon the sauce over the cooked shrimp.
10. Garnish with parsley and lemon.
11. Serve and enjoy!

Nutrition (Per Serving)

- Calories: 184
- Fat: 6g
- Carbohydrates: 6g
- Protein: 15g

Lemon and Garlic Scallops

Serving: 4
Prep Time: 10 minutes
Cook Time: 5 minutes
SmartPoints: 2
Ingredients:

- 1 tablespoon olive oil
- 1 ¼ pounds dried scallops
- 2 tablespoons all-purpose flour
- ¼ teaspoon sunflower seeds
- 4-5 garlic cloves, minced
- 1 scallion, chopped
- 1 pinch of ground sage
- 1 lemon juice
- 2 tablespoons parsley, chopped

Direction

1. Take a non-stick skillet and place over medium-high heat.

2. Add oil and allow the oil to heat up.
3. Take a medium sized bowl and add scallops alongside sunflower seeds and flour.
4. Place the scallops in the skillet and add scallions, garlic, and sage.
5. Sauté for 3-4 minutes until they show an opaque texture.
6. Stir in lemon juice and parsley.
7. Remove heat and serve hot!

Nutrition (Per Serving)

- Calories: 151
- Fat: 4g
- Carbohydrates: 10g
- Protein: 18g

Walnut Encrusted Salmon

Serving: 34
Prep Time: 10 minutes
Cook Time: 14 minutes
Ingredients:

- ½ cup walnuts
- 2 tablespoons stevia
- ½ tablespoon Dijon mustard
- ¼ teaspoon dill
- 2 salmon fillets (3 ounces each)
- 1 tablespoon olive oil
- Sunflower seeds and pepper to taste

How To:

1. Pre-heat your oven to 350 degrees F.
2. Add walnuts, mustard, stevia to food processor and process until your desired consistency is achieved.
3. Take a frying pan and place it over medium heat.
4. Add oil and let it heat up.
5. Add salmon and sear for 3 minutes.
6. Add walnut mix and coat well.
7. Transfer coated salmon to baking sheet, bake in oven for 8 minutes.
8. Serve and enjoy!

Nutrition (Per Serving)

- Calories: 373
- Fat: 43g
- Carbohydrates: 4g
- Protein: 20g

Roasted Lemon Swordfish

Serving: 4
Prep Time: 10 minutes
Cook Time: 70-80 minutes
Ingredients:

- ¼ cup parsley, chopped
- ½ teaspoon garlic, chopped
- ½ teaspoon canola oil
- 4 swordfish fillets, 6 ounces each
- ¼ teaspoon sunflower seeds
- 1 tablespoon sugar
- 2 lemons, quartered and seeds removed

How To:

1. Preheat your oven to 375 degrees F.
2. Take a small-sized bowl and add sugar, sunflower seeds, lemon wedges.
3. Toss well to coat them.
4. Take a shallow baking dish and add lemons, cover with aluminum foil.
5. Roast for about 60 minutes until lemons are tender and browned (Slightly).
6. Heat your grill and place the rack about 4 inches away from the source of heat.
7. Take a baking pan and coat it with cooking spray.
8. Transfer fish fillets to the pan and brush with oil on top spread garlic on top.
9. Grill for about 5 minutes each side until fillet turns opaque.
10. Transfer fish to a serving platter, squeeze roasted lemon on top.
11. Sprinkle parsley, serve with a lemon wedge on the side.
12. Enjoy!

Nutrition (Per Serving)

- Calories: 280
- Fat: 12g
- Net Carbohydrates: 4g
- Protein: 34g

Especial Glazed Salmon

Serving: 4
Prep Time: 45 minutes
Cook Time: 10 minutes
Ingredients:

- 4 pieces salmon fillets, 5 ounces each
- 4 tablespoons coconut aminos
- 4 teaspoon olive oil
- 2 teaspoons ginger, minced
- 4 teaspoons garlic, minced
- 2 tablespoons sugar-free ketchup
- 4 tablespoons dry white wine
- 2 tablespoons red boat fish sauce, low sodium

How To:

1. Take a bowl and mix in coconut aminos, garlic, ginger, fish sauce and mix.
2. Add salmon and let it marinate for 15-20 minutes.
3. Take a skillet/pan and place it over medium heat.
4. Add oil and let it heat up.
5. Add salmon fillets and cook on high heat for 3-4 minutes per side.
6. Remove dish once crispy.
7. Add sauce and wine.
8. Simmer for 5 minutes on low heat.
9. Return salmon to the glaze and flip until both sides are glazed.
10. Serve and enjoy!

Nutrition (Per Serving)

- Calories: 372
- Fat: 24g
- Carbohydrates: 3g
- Protein: 35g

Generous Stuffed Salmon Avocado

Serving: 2
Prep Time: 10 minutes
Cook Time: 30 minutes
Ingredients:

- 1 ripe organic avocado
- 2 ounces wild caught smoked salmon
- 1 ounce cashew cheese
- 2 tablespoons extra virgin olive oil
- Sunflower seeds as needed

How To:

1. Cut avocado in half and deseed.
2. Add the rest of the ingredients to a food processor and process until coarsely chopped.
3. Place mixture into avocado.
4. Serve and enjoy!

Nutrition (Per Serving)

- Calories: 525
- Fat: 48g
- Carbohydrates: 4g
- Protein: 19g

Spanish Mussels

Serving: 4
Prep Time: 10 minutes
Cook Time: 23 minutes
Ingredients:

- 3 tablespoons olive oil
- 2 pounds mussels, scrubbed
- Pepper to taste
- 3 cups canned tomatoes, crushed
- 1 shallot, chopped
- 2 garlic cloves, minced
- 2 cups low sodium vegetable stock
- 1/3 cup cilantro, chopped

How To:

1. Take a pan and place it over medium-high heat, add shallot and stir-cook for 3 minutes.
2. Add garlic, stock, tomatoes, pepper, stir and reduce heat, simmer for 10 minutes.
3. Add mussels, cilantro, and toss.
4. Cover and cook for 10 minutes more.
5. Serve and enjoy!

Nutrition (Per Serving)

- Calories: 210
- Fat: 2g
- Carbohydrates: 5g
- Protein: 8g

Tilapia Broccoli Platter

Serving: 2
Prep Time: 4 minutes
Cook Time: 14 minutes
Ingredients:

- 6 ounce tilapia, frozen
- 1 tablespoon almond butter
- 1 tablespoon garlic, minced
- 1 teaspoon lemon pepper seasoning
- 1 cup broccoli florets, fresh

How To:

1. Pre-heat your oven to 350 degrees F.
2. Add fish in aluminum foil packets.
3. Arrange broccoli around fish.
4. Sprinkle lemon pepper on top.
5. Close the packets and seal.
6. Bake for 14 minutes.
7. Take a bowl and add garlic and almond butter, mix well and keep the mixture on the side.
8. Remove the packet from oven and transfer to platter.
9. Place almond butter on top of the fish and broccoli, serve and enjoy!

Nutrition (Per Serving)

- Calories: 362
- Fat: 25g
- Carbohydrates: 2g
- Protein: 29g

Salmon with Peas and Parsley Dressing

Serving: 4
Prep Time: 15 minutes
Cook Time: 15 minutes
Ingredients:

- 16 ounces salmon fillets, boneless and skin-on
- 1 tablespoon parsley, chopped
- 10 ounces peas
- 9 ounces vegetable stock, low sodium
- 2 cups water
- ½ teaspoon oregano, dried
- ½ teaspoon sweet paprika
- 2 garlic cloves, minced
- A pinch of black pepper

How To:

1. Add garlic, parsley, paprika, oregano and stock to a food processor and blend.
2. Add water to your Instant Pot.
3. Add steam basket.
4. Add fish fillets inside the steamer basket.
5. Season with pepper.
6. Lock the lid and cook on HIGH pressure for 10 minutes.
7. Release the pressure naturally over 10 minutes .
8. Divide the fish amongst plates.
9. Add peas to the steamer basket and lock the lid again, cook on HIGH pressure for 5 minutes.
10. Quick release the pressure.
11. Divide the peas next to your fillets and serve with the parsley dressing drizzled on top

12. Enjoy!

Nutrition (Per Serving)

- Calories: 315
- Fat: 5g
- Carbohydrates: 14g
- Protein: 16g

Mackerel and Orange Medley

Serving: 4
Prep Time: 10 minutes
Cook Time: 10 minutes
Ingredients:

- 4 mackerel fillets, skinless and boneless
- 4 spring onion, chopped
- 1 teaspoon olive oil
- 1-inch ginger piece, grated
- Black pepper as needed
- Juice and zest of 1 whole orange
- 1 cup low sodium fish stock

How To:

1. Season the fillets with black pepper and rub olive oil.
2. Add stock, orange juice, ginger, orange zest and onion to Instant Pot.
3. Place a steamer basket and add the fillets.
4. Lock the lid and cook on HIGH pressure for 10 minutes.
5. Release the pressure naturally over 10 minutes.
6. Divide the fillets amongst plates and drizzle the orange sauce from the pot over the fish.
7. Enjoy!

Nutrition (Per Serving)

- Calories: 200
- Fat: 4g
- Carbohydrates: 19g
- Protein: 14g

Spicy Chili Salmon

Serving: 4
Prep Time: 10 minutes
Cook Time: 7 minutes
Ingredients:

- 4 salmon fillets, boneless and skin-on
- 2 tablespoons assorted chili peppers, chopped
- Juice of 1 lemon
- 1 lemon, sliced
- 1 cup water
- Black pepper

How To:

1. Add water to the Instant Pot.
2. Add steamer basket and add salmon fillets, season the fillets with salt and pepper.
3. Drizzle lemon juice on top.
4. Top with lemon slices.
5. Lock the lid and cook on HIGH pressure for 7 minutes.
6. Release the pressure naturally over 10 minutes.
7. Divide the salmon and lemon slices between serving plates.
8. Enjoy!

Nutrition (Per Serving)

- Calories: 281
- Fats: 8g
- Carbs: 19g
- Protein:7g

Simple One Pot Mussels

Serving: 4
Prep Time: 10 minutes
Cook Time: 5 minutes
Ingredients:

- 2 tablespoons butter
- 2 chopped shallots
- 4 minced garlic cloves
- ½ cup broth
- ½ cup white wine
- 2 pounds cleaned mussels
- Lemon and parsley for serving

How To:

1. Clean the mussels and remove the beard.
2. Discard any mussels that do not close when tapped against a hard surface.
3. Set your pot to Sauté mode and add chopped onion and butter.
4. Stir and sauté onions.
5. Add garlic and cook for 1 minute.
6. Add broth and wine.
7. Lock the lid and cook for 5 minutes on HIGH pressure.
8. Release the pressure naturally over 10 minutes.
9. Serve with a sprinkle of parsley and enjoy!

Nutrition (Per Serving)

- Calories: 286
- Fats: 14g
- Carbs: 12g
- Protein: 28g

Lemon Pepper and Salmon

Serving: 3
Prep Time: 5 minute
Cook Time: 6 minutes
Ingredients:

- ¾ cup water
- Few sprigs of parsley, basil, tarragon, basil
- 1 pound of salmon, skin on
- 3 teaspoons ghee
- ¼ teaspoon salt
- ½ teaspoon pepper
- ½ lemon, thinly sliced
- 1 whole carrot, julienned

How To:
1. Set your pot to Sauté mode and water and herbs.
2. Place a steamer rack inside your pot and place salmon.
3. Drizzle the ghee on top of the salmon and season with salt and pepper.
4. Cover lemon slices.
5. Lock the lid and cook on HIGH pressure for 3 minutes.
6. Release the pressure naturally over 10 minutes.
7. Transfer the salmon to a serving platter.
8. Set your pot to Sauté mode and add vegetables.
9. Cook for 1-2 minutes.
10. Serve with vegetables and salmon.
11. Enjoy!

Nutrition (Per Serving)

- Calories: 464
- Fat: 34g
- Carbohydrates: 3g
- Protein: 34g

Simple Sautéed Garlic and Parsley Scallops
Serving: 4
Prep Time: 5 minutes
Cook Time: 25 minutes
Ingredients:

- 8 tablespoons almond butter
- 2 garlic cloves, minced
- 16 large sea scallops
- Sunflower seeds and pepper to taste
- 1 ½ tablespoons olive oil

How To:
1. Seasons scallops with sunflower seeds and pepper.
2. Take a skillet, place it over medium heat, add oil and let it heat up.
3. Sauté scallops for 2 minutes per side, repeat until all scallops are cooked.
4. Add almond butter to the skillet and let it melt.
5. Stir in garlic and cook for 15 minutes.
6. Return scallops to skillet and stir to coat.
7. Serve and enjoy!

Nutrition (Per Serving)

- Calories: 417
- Fat: 31g
- Net Carbohydrates: 5g
- Protein: 29g

Salmon and Cucumber Platter

Serving: 4
Prep Time: 10 minutes
Cook Time: nil
Ingredients:

- 2 cucumbers, cubed
- 2 teaspoons fresh squeezed lemon juice
- 4 ounces non-fat yogurt
- 1 teaspoon lemon zest, grated
- Pepper to taste
- 2 teaspoons dill, chopped
- 8 ounces smoked salmon, flaked

How To:

1. Take a bowl and add cucumbers, lemon juice, lemon zest, pepper, dill, salmon, yogurt and toss well.
2. Serve cold.
3. Enjoy!

Nutrition (Per Serving)

- Calories: 242
- Fat: 3g
- Carbohydrates: 3g
- Protein: 3g

Tuna Paté

Serving: 4
Prep Time: 10 minutes
Cook Time: nil
Ingredients:

- 6 ounces canned tuna, drained and flaked
- 3 teaspoons fresh lemon juice
- 1 teaspoon onion, minced
- 8 ounces low-fat cream cheese
- ¼ cup parsley, chopped

How To:

1. Take a bowl and mix in tuna, cream cheese, lemon juice, parsley, onion and stir well.
2. Serve cold and enjoy!

Nutrition (Per Serving)

- Calories: 172
- Fat: 2g
- Carbohydrates: 8g
- Protein: 4g

Cinnamon Salmon

Serving: 4
Prep Time: 10 minutes
Cook Time: 10 minutes
Ingredients:

- 2 salmon fillets, boneless and skin on
- Pepper to taste
- 1 tablespoon cinnamon powder
- 1 tablespoon organic olive oil

How To:

1. Take a pan and place it over medium heat, add oil and let it heat up.
2. Add pepper, cinnamon and stir.
3. Add salmon, skin side up and cook for 5 minutes on both sides.
4. Divide between plates and serve.
5. Enjoy!

Nutrition (Per Serving)

- Calories: 220
- Fat: 8g
- Carbohydrates: 11g
- Protein: 8g

Scallop and Strawberry Mix

Serving: 4
Prep Time: 10 minutes
Cook Time: 6 minutes
Ingredients:

- 4 ounces scallops
- ½ cup Pico De Gallo
- ½ cup strawberries, chopped
- 1 tablespoon lime juice
- Pepper to taste

How To:

1. Take a pan and place it over medium heat, add scallops and cook for 3 minutes on both sides.
2. Remove heat.
3. Take a bowl and add strawberries, lime juice, Pico De Gallo, scallops, pepper and toss well.
4. Serve and enjoy!

Nutrition (Per Serving)

- Calories: 169
- Fat: 2g
- Carbohydrates: 8g
- Protein: 13g

Salmon and Orange Dish

Serving: 4
Prep Time: 10 minute
Cook Time: 15 minutes
Ingredients:

- 4 salmon fillets
- 1 cup orange juice
- 2 tablespoons arrowroot and water mixture
- 1 teaspoon orange peel, grated
- 1 teaspoon black pepper

How To:

1. Add the listed ingredients to your pot.
2. Lock the lid and cook on HIGH pressure for 12 minutes.
3. Release the pressure naturally.
4. Serve and enjoy!

Nutrition (Per Serving)

- Calories:583
- Fat: 20g
- Carbohydrates: 71g
- Protein: 33g

Mesmerizing Coconut Haddock

Serving: 3
Prep Time: 10 minutes
Cook Time: 12 minutes
Ingredients:

- 4 haddock fillets, 5 ounces each, boneless
- 2 tablespoons coconut oil, melted
- 1 cup coconut, shredded and unsweetened
- ¼ cup hazelnuts, ground
- Sunflower seeds to taste

How To:

1. Pre-heat your oven to 400 degrees F.
2. Line a baking sheet with parchment paper.
3. Keep it on the side.
4. Pat fish fillets with paper towel and season with sunflower seeds.
5. Take a bowl and stir in hazelnuts and shredded coconut.
6. Drag fish fillets through the coconut mix until both sides are coated well.
7. Transfer to baking dish.
8. Brush with coconut oil.
9. Bake for about 12 minutes until flaky.
10. Serve and enjoy!

Nutrition (Per Serving)

- Calories: 299
- Fat: 24g
- Carbohydrates: 1g
- Protein: 20g

Asparagus and Lemon Salmon Dish

Serving: 3
Prep Time: 5 minutes
Cook Time: 15 minutes
Ingredients:

- 2 salmon fillets, 6 ounces each, skin on
- Sunflower seeds to taste
- 1 pound asparagus, trimmed
- 2 cloves garlic, minced
- 3 tablespoons almond butter
- ¼ cup cashew cheese

How To:

1. Pre-heat your oven to 400 degrees F.
2. Line a baking sheet with oil.
3. Take a kitchen towel and pat your salmon dry, season as needed.
4. Put salmon onto the baking sheet and arrange asparagus around it.
5. Place a pan over medium heat and melt almond butter.
6. Add garlic and cook for 3 minutes until garlic browns slightly.
7. Drizzle sauce over salmon.
8. Sprinkle salmon with cheese and bake for 12 minutes until salmon looks cooked all the way and is flaky.
9. Serve and enjoy!

Nutrition (Per Serving)

- Calories: 434
- Fat: 26g
- Carbohydrates: 6g
- Protein: 42g

Ecstatic "Foiled" Fish

Serving: 4
Prep Time: 20 minutes
Cook Time: 40 minutes
Ingredients:

- 2 rainbow trout fillets
- 1 tablespoon olive oil
- 2 teaspoon garlic salt
- 1 teaspoon ground black pepper
- 1 fresh jalapeno pepper, sliced
- 1 lemon, sliced

How To:

1. Pre-heat your oven to 400 degrees F.
2. Rinse your fish and pat them dry.
3. Rub the fillets with olive oil, season with some garlic salt and black pepper.
4. Place each of your seasoned fillets on a large sized sheet of aluminum foil.
5. Top it with some jalapeno slices and squeeze the juice from your lemons over your fish.
6. Arrange the lemon slices on top of your fillets.
7. Carefully seal up the edges of your foil and form a nice enclosed packet.
8. Place your packets on your baking sheet.
9. Bake them for about 20 minutes.
10. Once the flakes start to flake off with a fork, the fish is ready!

Nutrition (Per Serving)

- Calories: 213
- Fat: 10g
- Carbohydrates: 8g
- Protein: 24g

Brazilian Shrimp Stew

Serving: 4
Prep Time: 20 minutes
Cook Time: 25 minutes
Ingredients:

- 4 tablespoons lime juice
- 1 ½ tablespoons cumin, ground
- 1 ½ tablespoons paprika
- 2 ½ teaspoons garlic, minced
- 1 ½ teaspoons pepper
- 2 pounds tilapia fillets, cut into bits
- 1 large onion, chopped
- 3 large bell peppers, cut into strips
- 1 can (14 ounces) tomato, drained
- 1 can (14 ounces) coconut milk
- Handful of cilantro, chopped

How To:

1. Take a large sized bowl and add lime juice, cumin, paprika, garlic, pepper and mix well.
2. Add tilapia and coat it up.
3. Cover and allow to marinate for 20 minutes.
4. Set your Instant Pot to Saute mode(HIGH) and add olive oil.
5. Add onions and cook for 3 minutes until tender.
6. Add pepper strips, tilapia, and tomatoes to a skillet.
7. Pour coconut milk and cover, simmer for 20 minutes.
8. Add cilantro during the final few minutes.
9. Serve and enjoy!

Nutrition (Per Serving)

- Calories: 471
- Fat: 44g
- Carbohydrates: 13g
- Protein: 12g

Inspiring Cajun Snow Crab

Serving: 2
Prep Time: 10 minutes
Cook Time: 10 minutes
Ingredients:

- 1 lemon, fresh and quartered
- 3 tablespoons Cajun seasoning
- 2 bay leaves
- 4 snow crab legs, precooked and defrosted
- Golden ghee

How To:

1. Take a large pot and fill it about halfway with sunflower seeds and water.
2. Bring the water to a boil.
3. Squeeze lemon juice into the pot and toss in remaining lemon quarters.
4. Add bay leaves and Cajun seasoning.
5. Season for 1 minute.
6. Add crab legs and boil for 8 minutes (make sure to keep them submerged the whole time).
7. Melt ghee in microwave and use as dipping sauce, enjoy!

Nutrition (Per Serving)

- Calories: 643
- Fat: 51g
- Carbohydrates: 3g
- Protein: 41g

Grilled Lime Shrimp

Serving: 8
Prep Time: 25 minutes
Cook Time: 5 minutes
Ingredients:

- 1 pound medium shrimp, peeled and deveined
- 1 lime, juiced
- ½ cup olive oil
- 3 tablespoons Cajun seasoning

How To:

1. Take a re-sealable zip bag and add lime juice, Cajun seasoning, olive oil.
2. Add shrimp and shake it well, let it marinate for 20 minutes.
3. Pre-heat your outdoor grill to medium heat.
4. Lightly grease the grate.
5. Remove shrimp from marinade and cook for 2 minutes per side.
6. Serve and enjoy!

Nutrition (Per Serving)

- Calories: 188
- Fat: 3g
- Net Carbohydrates: 1.2g
- Protein: 13g

Calamari Citrus

Serving: 4
Prep Time: 10 minutes
Cook Time: 5 minutes
Ingredients:

- 1 lime, sliced
- 1 lemon, sliced
- 2 pounds calamari tubes and tentacles, sliced
- Pepper to taste
- ¼ cup olive oil
- 2 garlic cloves, minced
- 3 tablespoons lemon juice
- 1 orange, peeled and cut into segments
- 2 tablespoons cilantro, chopped

How To:

1. Take a bowl and add calamari, pepper, lime slices, lemon slices, orange slices, garlic, oil, cilantro, lemon juice and toss well.
2. Take a pan and place it over medium-high heat.
3. Add calamari mix and cook for 5 minutes.
4. Divide into bowls and serve.
5. Enjoy!

Nutrition (Per Serving)

- Calories: 190
- Fat: 2g
- Net Carbohydrates: 11g
- Protein: 14g

Spiced Up Salmon

Serving: 4
Prep Time: 10 minutes
Cook Time: 10 minutes
Ingredients:

- 4 salmon fillets
- 2 tablespoons olive oil
- 1 teaspoon cumin, ground
- 1 teaspoon sweet paprika
- 1 teaspoon chili powder
- ½ teaspoon garlic powder
- Pinch of pepper

How To:

1. Take a bowl and add cumin, paprika, onion, chili powder, garlic powder, pepper and toss well.
2. Rub the salmon in the mixture.
3. Take a pan and place it over medium heat, add oil and let it heat up.
4. Add salmon and cook for 5 minutes, both sides.
5. Divide between plates and serve.
6. Enjoy!

Nutrition (Per Serving)

- Calories: 220
- Fat: 10g
- Net Carbohydrates: 8g
- Protein: 10g

Coconut Cream Shrimp

Serving: 4
Prep Time: 10 minutes
Cook Time: nil
Ingredients:

- 1 pound shrimp, cooked , peeled and deveined
- 1 tablespoon coconut cream
- ¼ teaspoon jalapeno, chopped
- ½ teaspoon lime juice
- 1 tablespoon parsley, chopped
- Pinch of pepper

How To:

1. Take a bowl and add shrimp, cream, jalapeno, lime juice, parsley, pepper.
2. Toss well and divide into small bowls.
3. Serve and enjoy!

Nutrition (Per Serving)

- Calories: 183
- Fat: 5g
- Net Carbohydrates: 12g
- Protein: 8g

Shrimp and Avocado Platter

Serving: 8
Prep Time: 10 minutes
Cook Time: nil
Ingredients:

- 2 green onions, chopped
- 2 avocados, pitted, peeled and cut into chunks
- 2 tablespoons cilantro, chopped
- 1 cup shrimp, cooked, peeled and deveined
- Pinch of pepper

How To:

1. Take a bowl and add cooked shrimp, avocado, green onions, cilantro, pepper.
2. Toss well and serve.
3. Enjoy!

Nutrition (Per Serving)

- Calories: 160
- Fat: 2g
- Net Carbohydrates: 5g
- Protein: 6g

Calamari

Serving: 4
Prep Time: 10 minutes +1 hour marinating
Cook Time: 8 minutes
Ingredients:

- 2 tablespoons extra virgin olive oil
- 1 teaspoon chili powder
- ½ teaspoon ground cumin
- Zest of 1 lime
- Juice of 1 lime
- Dash of sea sunflower seeds
- 1 ½ pounds squid, cleaned and split open, with tentacles cut into ½ inch rounds
- 2 tablespoons cilantro, chopped
- 2 tablespoons red bell pepper, minced

How To:

1. Take a medium bowl and stir in olive oil, chili powder, cumin, lime zest, sea sunflower seeds, lime juice and pepper.
2. Add squid and let it marinade and stir to coat, coat and let it refrigerate for 1 hour
3. Pre-heat your oven to broil.
4. Arrange squid on a baking sheet, broil for 8 minutes turn once until tender.
5. Garnish the broiled calamari with cilantro and red bell pepper.
6. Serve and enjoy!

Nutrition (Per Serving)

- Calories: 159
- Fat: 13g
- Carbohydrates: 12g
- Protein: 3g

Hearty Deep Fried Prawn and Rice Croquettes

Serving: 8
Prep Time: 25 minute
Cook Time: 13 minutes
Ingredients:

- 2 tablespoons almond butter
- ½ onion, chopped
- 4 ounces shrimp, peeled and chopped
- 2 tablespoons all-purpose flour
- 1 tablespoon white wine
- ½ cup almond milk
- 2 tablespoons almond milk
- 2 cups cooked rice
- 1 tablespoon parmesan, grated
- 1 teaspoon fresh dill, chopped
- 1 teaspoon sunflower seeds
- Ground pepper as needed
- Vegetable oil for frying
- 3 tablespoons all-purpose flour
- 1 whole egg
- ½ cup breadcrumbs

How To:

1. Take a large skillet and place it over medium heat, add almond butter and let it melt.
2. Add onion, cook and stir for 5 minutes.
3. Add shrimp and cook for 1-2 minutes.
4. Stir in 2 tablespoons flour, white wine, pour in almond milk gradually and cook for 3-5 minutes until the sauce thickens.
5. Remove white sauce from heat and stir in rice, mix evenly.
6. Add parmesan, cheese, dill, sunflower seeds, pepper and let it cool for 15 minutes.
7. Heat oil in large saucepan and bring it to 350 degrees F.
8. Take a bowl and whisk in egg, spread breadcrumbs on a plate.
9. Form rice mixture into 8 balls and roll 1 ball in flour, dip in egg and coat with crumbs, repeat with all balls.
10. Deep fry balls for 3 minutes.
11. Enjoy!

Nutrition (Per Serving)

- Calories: 182
- Fat: 7g
- Carbohydrates: 21g
- Protein: 7g

Easy Garlic Almond butter Shrimp

Serving: 4
Prep Time: 15 minutes
Cook Time: 30 minutes
Ingredients:

- 4 pounds shrimp
- 1-2 tablespoons garlic, minced
- ½ cup almond butter
- 1 tablespoon lemon pepper seasoning
- ½ teaspoon garlic powder

How To:

1. Pre-heat your oven to 300 degrees F.
2. Take a bowl and mix in garlic and almond butter.
3. Place shrimp in a pan and dot with almond butter garlic mix.
4. Sprinkle garlic powder and lemon pepper.
5. Bake for 30 minutes.

6. Enjoy!

Nutrition (Per Serving)

- Calories: 749
- Fat: 30g
- Net Carbohydrates: 7g
- Protein: 74g

Blackened Tilapia

Serving: 2
Prep Time: 9 minutes
Cook Time: 9 minutes
Ingredients:

- 1 cup cauliflower, chopped
- 1 teaspoon red pepper flakes
- 1 tablespoon Italian seasoning
- 1 tablespoon garlic, minced
- 6 ounces tilapia
- 1 cup English cucumber, chopped with peel
- 2 tablespoons olive oil
- 1 sprig dill, chopped
- 1 teaspoon stevia
- 3 tablespoons lime juice
- 2 tablespoons Cajun blackened seasoning

How To:

1. Take a bowl and add the seasoning ingredients (except Cajun).
2. Add a tablespoon of oil and whip.
3. Pour dressing over cauliflower and cucumber.
4. Brush the fish with olive oil on both sides.
5. Take a skillet and grease it well with 1 tablespoon of olive oil.
6. Press Cajun seasoning on both sides of fish.
7. Cook fish for 3 minutes per side.
8. Serve with vegetables and enjoy!

Nutrition (Per Serving)

- Calories: 530
- Fat: 33g
- Net Carbohydrates: 4g
- Protein: 32g

Light Lobster Bisque

Serving: 4
Prep Time: 10 minutes
400 Cook Time: 6 minutes
Ingredients:

- 1 cup diced carrots
- 1 cup diced celery
- 29 ounces diced tomatoes
- 2 minced whole shallots
- 1 clove of minced garlic
- 1 tablespoon butter
- 32 ounce chicken broth, low-sodium
- 1 teaspoon dill, dried
- 1 teaspoon freshly ground black pepper
- ½ teaspoon paprika
- 4 lobster tails
- 1 pint heavy whipping cream

How To:

1. Add butter, garlic and minced shallots to a microwave safe bowl.
2. Microwave for 2-3 minutes on HIGH.
3. Add tomatoes, celery, carrot, minced shallots, garlic to your Instant Pot.
4. Add chicken broth and spices to the Pot.
5. Use a knife to cut the lobster tails if you prefer and add them to the Instant Pot.
6. Lock the lid and cook on HIGH pressure for 4 minutes.
7. Release the pressure naturally over 10 minutes.
8. Use an immersion blender to puree to your desired chunkiness.
9. Serve and enjoy!

Nutrition (Per Serving)

- Calories: 437
- Fats: 17g
- Carbs: 21g
- Protein: 38g

Herbal Shrimp Risotto

Serving: 4
Prep Time: 10 minutes
Cook Time: 8 minutes
Ingredients:

- 2 pounds shrimp with their tails removed
- 1 cup instant rice
- 2 cups vegetable broth
- 1 chopped up onion
- 1 cup chicken breast cut into fine strips
- ¼ cup lemon juice
- 1 teaspoon crushed red pepper
- ¼ cup parsley
- ¼ cup fresh dill
- 6 pieces chopped up garlic cloves
- 1 tablespoon black pepper
- ½ cup parmesan
- 1 cup mozzarella cheese

How To:

1. Add the listed ingredients to your Instant Pot and stir.
2. Lock the lid and cook on HIGH pressure for 8 minutes.
3. Release the pressure naturally over 10 minutes.
4. Open lid and top with cheese.
5. Serve hot and enjoy!

Nutrition (Per Serving)

- Calories: 463
- Fat: 8g
- Carbohydrates: 63g
- Protein: 29g

Thai Pumpkin Seafood Stew

Serving: 4

Prep Time: 5 minutes

Cook Time: 35 minutes

Ingredients:

- 1 ½ tablespoons fresh galangal, chopped
- 1 teaspoon lime zest
- 1 small kabocha squash
- 32 medium sized mussels, fresh
- 1 pound shrimp
- 16 thai leaves
- 1 can coconut milk
- 1 tablespoon lemongrass, minced
- 4 garlic cloves, roughly chopped
- 32 medium clams, fresh
- 1 ½ pounds fresh salmon
- 2 tablespoons coconut oil
- Pepper to taste

How To:

1. Add coconut milk, lemongrass, galangal, garlic, lime leaves in a small-sized saucepan, bring to a boil.
2. Let it simmer for 25 minutes.
3. Strain mixture through a fine sieve into the large soup pot and bring to a simmer.
4. Add oil to a pan and heat up, add Kabocha squash.
5. Season with salt and pepper, sauté for 5 minutes.
6. Add mix to coconut mix.
7. Heat oil in a pan and add fish shrimp, season with salt and pepper, cook for 4 minutes.
8. Add mixture to coconut milk, mix alongside clams and mussels.
9. Simmer for 8 minutes, garnish with basil and enjoy!

Nutrition (Per Serving)

- Calories: 370
- Fat: 16g
- Net Carbohydrates: 10g
- Protein: 16g

Pistachio Sole Fish

Serving: 4

Prep Time: 5 minutes

Cook Time: 10 minutes

Ingredients:

- 4 (5 ounces) boneless sole fillets
- Sunflower seeds and pepper as needed
- ½ cup pistachios, finely chopped
- Juice of 1 lemon
- 1 teaspoon extra virgin olive oil

How To:

1. Pre-heat your oven to 350 degrees F.
2. Line a baking sheet with parchment paper and keep it on the side.
3. Pat fish dry with kitchen towels and lightly season with sunflower seeds and pepper.
4. Take a small bowl and stir in pistachios.
5. Place sole on the prepared baking sheet and press 2 tablespoons of pistachio mixture on top of each fillet.
6. Drizzle fish with lemon juice and olive oil.
7. Bake for 10 minutes until the top is golden and fish flakes with a fork.
8. Serve and enjoy!

Nutrition (Per Serving)

- Calories: 166
- Fat: 6g
- Carbohydrates: 2g
- Protein: 26g

Chapter 9: Salad Recipes

Spring Salad

Serving: 2
Prep Time: 10-15 minutes
Cook Time: 0 minutes
Ingredients:

- 2 ounces mixed green vegetables
- 3 tablespoons roasted pine nuts
- 2 tablespoons 5 minute 5 Keto Raspberry Vinaigrette
- 2 tablespoons shaved Parmesan
- 2 slices bacon
- Pepper as required

How To:

1. Take a cooking pan and add bacon, cook the bacon until crispy.
2. Take a bowl and add the salad ingredients and mix well, add crumbled bacon into the salad.
3. Mix well.
4. Dress it with your favorite dressing.
5. Enjoy!

Nutrition (Per Serving)

- Calories: 209
- Fat: 17g
- Net Carbohydrates: 10g
- Protein: 4g

Hearty Orange and Onion Salad

Serving: 2
Prep Time: 10 minutes
Cook Time: nil
Ingredients:

- 6 large oranges
- 3 tablespoons red wine vinegar
- 6 tablespoons olive oil
- 1 teaspoon dried oregano
- 1 red onion, thinly sliced
- 1 cup olive oil
- ¼ cup fresh chives, chopped
- Ground black pepper

How To:

1. Peel orange and cut into 4-5 crosswise slices.
2. Transfer orange to shallow dish.
3. Drizzle vinegar, olive oil on top.
4. Sprinkle oregano.
5. Toss well to mix.
6. Chill for 30 minutes and arrange sliced onion and black olives on top.
7. Sprinkle more chives and pepper.
8. Serve and enjoy!

Nutrition (Per Serving)

- Calories: 120
- Fat: 6g
- Carbohydrates: 20g
- Protein: 2g

Ground Beef Bell Peppers

Serving: 3
Prep Time: 10 minutes
Cook Time: 10 minutes
Ingredients:

- 1 onion, chopped
- 2 tablespoons coconut oil
- 1 pound ground beef
- 1 red bell pepper, diced
- 2 cups spinach, chopped
- Pepper to taste

How To:

1. Take a skillet and place it over medium heat.
2. Add onion and cook until slightly browned.
3. Add spinach and ground beef.
4. Stir fry until done.
5. Take the mixture and fill up the bell peppers.
6. Serve and enjoy!

Nutrition (Per Serving)

- Calories: 350
- Fat: 23g
- Carbohydrates: 4g
- Protein: 28g

Healthy Mediterranean Lamb Chops

Serving: 4
Prep Time: 10 minutes
Cook Time: 10 minute
Ingredients:

- 4 lamb shoulder chops, 8 ounces each
- 2 tablespoons Dijon mustard
- 2 tablespoons Balsamic vinegar
- ½ cup olive oil
- 2 tablespoons shredded fresh basil

How To:

1. Pat your lamb chops dry using a kitchen towel and arrange them on a shallow glass baking dish.
2. Take a bowl and whisk in Dijon mustard, balsamic vinegar, pepper and mix them well.
3. Whisk in the oil very slowly into the marinade until the mixture is smooth.
4. Stir in basil.
5. Pour the marinade over the lamb chops and stir to coat both sides well .
6. Cover the chops and allow them to marinate for 1-4 hours (chilled).
7. Take the chops out and let them rest for 30 minutes to allow the temperature to reach a normal level.
8. Pre-heat your grill to medium heat and add oil to the grate.
9. Grill the lamb chops for 5-10 minutes per side until both sides are browned.
10. Once the center reads 145 degrees F, the chops are ready, serve and enjoy!

Nutrition (Per Serving)

- Calories: 521
- Fat: 45g
- Carbohydrates: 3.5g
- Protein: 22g

A Turtle Friend Salad

Serving: 6
Prep Time: 5 minutes
Cook Time: 5 minutes
SmartPoints: 1
Ingredients:

- 1 Romaine lettuce, chopped
- 3 Roma tomatoes, diced
- 1 English cucumber, diced
- 1 small red onion, diced
- ½ cup parsley, chopped
- 2 tablespoons virgin olive oil
- ½ large lemon, juice
- 1 teaspoon garlic powder
- Sunflower seeds and pepper to taste

How To:

1. Wash the vegetables thoroughly under cold water.
2. Prepare them by chopping, dicing or mincing as needed.
3. Take a large salad bowl and transfer the prepped veggies.
4. Add vegetable oil, olive oil, lemon juice, and spice.
5. Toss well to coat.
6. Serve chilled if preferred.
7. Enjoy!

Nutrition (Per Serving)

- Calories: 200
- Fat: 8g
- Carbohydrates: 18g
- Protein: 10g

Avocado and Cilantro Mix

Serving: 2
Prep Time: 10 minutes
Cook Time: nil
Ingredients:

- 2 avocados, peeled, pitted and diced
- 1 sweet onion, chopped
- 1 green bell pepper, chopped
- 1 large ripe tomato, chopped
- ¼ cup of fresh cilantro, chopped
- ½ lime, juiced
- Sunflower seeds and pepper as needed

How To:

1. Take a medium sized bowl and add onion, tomato, avocados, bell pepper, lime and cilantro.
2. Give the whole mixture a toss.
3. Season accordingly and serve chilled.
4. Enjoy!

Nutrition (Per Serving)

- Calories: 126
- Fat: 10g
- Carbohydrates: 10g
- Protein: 2g

Exceptional Watercress and Melon Salad

Serving: 4
Prep Time: 15 minutes
Cook Time: 20 minutes
Ingredients:

- 3 tablespoons lime juice
- 1 teaspoon date paste
- 1 teaspoon fresh ginger root, minced
- ¼ cup vegetable oil
- 2 bunch watercress, chopped
- 2 ½ cups watermelon, cubed
- 2 ½ cups cantaloupe, cubed
- 1/3 cup almonds, toasted and sliced

How To:

1. Take a large sized bowl and add lime juice, ginger, date paste.
2. Whisk well and add oil.
3. Season with pepper and sunflower seeds.
4. Add watercress, watermelon.
5. Toss well
6. Transfer to a serving bowl and garnish with sliced almonds.
7. Enjoy!

Nutrition (Per Serving)

- Calories: 274
- Fat: 20g
- Carbohydrates: 21g
- Protein: 7g

Zucchini and Onions Platter

Serving: 4
Prep Time: 15 minutes
Cook Time: 45 minutes
Ingredients:

- 3 large zucchini, julienned
- 1 cup cherry tomatoes, halved
- ½ cup basil
- 2 red onions, thinly sliced
- ¼ teaspoon sunflower seeds
- 1 teaspoon cayenne pepper
- 2 tablespoons lemon juice

How To:

1. Create zucchini Zoodles by using a vegetable peeler and shaving the zucchini with peeler lengthwise until you get to the core and seeds.
2. Turn zucchini and repeat until you have long strips.
3. Discard seeds.
4. Lay strips in cutting board and slice lengthwise to your desired thickness.
5. Mix Zoodles in a bowl alongside onion, basil, tomatoes and toss.
6. Sprinkle sunflower seeds and cayenne pepper on top.
7. Drizzle lemon juice.
8. Serve and enjoy!

Nutrition (Per Serving)

- Calories: 156
- Fat: 8g
- Carbohydrates: 6g
- Protein: 7g

Tender Watermelon and Radish Salad

Serving: 4
Prep Time: 15 minutes
Cook Time: 25 minutes
Ingredients:

- 10 medium beets, peeled and cut into 1-inch chunks
- 1 teaspoon extra virgin olive oil
- 4 cups seedless watermelon, diced
- 1 tablespoon fresh thyme, chopped
- 1 lemon, juiced
- 2 cups kale, torn
- 3 cups radish, diced
- Sunflower seeds, to taste
- Pepper, to taste

How To:

1. Pre-heat your oven to 350 degrees F.
2. Take a small bowl and add beets, olive oil and toss well to coat the beets.
3. Roast beets for 25 minutes until tender.
4. Transfer to large bowl and cool them.
5. Add watermelon, kale, radishes, thyme, lemon juice, and toss.
6. Season sea sunflower seeds and pepper.
7. Serve and enjoy!

Nutrition (Per Serving)

- Calories: 178
- Fat: 2g
- Carbohydrates: 39g
- Protein: 6g

Fiery Tomato Salad

Serving: 4
Prep Time: 10 minutes
Cook Time: 25 minutes
Ingredients:

- ½ cup scallions, chopped
- 1 pound cherry tomatoes
- 3 teaspoons olive oil
- Sea sunflower seeds and freshly ground black pepper, to taste
- 1 tablespoon red wine vinegar

How To:

1. Season tomatoes with spices and oil.
2. Heat your oven to 450 degrees F.
3. Take a baking sheet and spread the tomatoes.
4. Bake for 15 minutes.
5. Stir and turn the tomatoes.
6. Then, bake again for 10 minutes.
7. Take a bowl and mix the roasted tomatoes with all the remaining ingredients.
8. Serve and enjoy!

Nutrition (Per Serving)

- Calories: 115
- Fat: 10.4g
- Carbohydrates: 5.4g
- Protein: 12g

Healthy Cauliflower Salad

Serving: 4
Prep Time: 10 minutes
Cook Time: nil
Ingredients:

- 1 head cauliflower, broken into florets
- 1 small onion, chopped
- 1/8 cup extra virgin olive oil
- ¼ cup apple cider vinegar
- ½ teaspoon sea salt
- ½ teaspoon black pepper
- ¼ cup dried cranberries
- ¼ cup pumpkin seeds

How To:

1. Wash the cauliflower thoroughly and break down into florets.
2. Transfer the florets to a bowl.
3. Take another bowl and whisk in oil, salt, pepper and vinegar.
4. Add pumpkin seeds, cranberries to the bowl with dressing.
5. Mix well and pour dressing over cauliflower florets.
6. Toss well.
7. Add onions and toss.
8. Chill and serve.
9. Enjoy!

Nutrition (Per Serving)

- Calories: 163
- Fat: 11g
- Carbohydrates: 16g
- Protein: 3g

Chickpea Salad

Serving: 4
Prep Time: 6 minutes
Cook Time: Nil
Ingredients:

- 1 cup canned chickpeas, drained and rinsed.
- 2 spring onions, thinly sliced.
- 1 small cucumber, diced.
- 2 green bell peppers, chopped.
- 2 tomatoes, diced.
- 2 tablespoons fresh parsley, chopped.
- 1 teaspoon capers, drained and rinsed.
- Half a lemon, juiced.
- 2 tablespoons sunflower oil.
- 1 tablespoon red wine vinegar.
- Pinch of dried oregano.
- Sunflower seeds and pepper to taste

How To:

1. Take a medium sized bowl and add chickpeas, spring onions, cucumber, bell pepper, tomato, parsley and capers.
2. Take another bowl and mix in the rest of the ingredients, pour mixture over chickpea salad and toss well.
3. Coat and serve, enjoy!

Nutrition (Per Serving)

- Calories: 74
- Fat: 0.7g
- Carbohydrates: 16g
- Protein: 2g

Dashing Bok Choy Samba

Serving: 3
Prep Time: 5 minutes
Cook Time: 15 minutes
Ingredients:

- 4 bok choy, sliced
- 1 onion, sliced
- ½ cup Parmesan cheese, grated
- 4 teaspoons coconut cream
- Sunflower seeds and freshly ground black pepper, to taste

How To:

1. Mix bok choy with black pepper and sunflower seeds.
2. Take a cooking pan, heat the oil and to sauté sliced onion for 5 minutes.
3. Then add cream and seasoned bok choy.
4. Cook for 6 minutes.
5. Stir in Parmesan cheese and cover with a lid.
6. Reduce the heat to low and cook for 3 minutes.
7. Serve warm and enjoy!

Nutrition (Per Serving)

- Calories: 112
- Fat: 4.9g
- Carbohydrates: 1.9g
- Protein: 3g

Simple Avocado Caprese Salad

Serving: 6
Prep Time: 15 minutes
Cook Time: 29 minutes
Ingredients:

- 2 avocados, cubed
- 1 cup cherry tomatoes, halved
- 8 ounces mozzarella balls, halved
- 2 tablespoons finely chopped fresh basil
- 2 tablespoons olive oil
- 2 tablespoons balsamic vinegar
- 1 tablespoon sunflower seeds
- Fresh ground black pepper

How To:

1. Take a bowl and add the listed ingredients, toss them well until thoroughly mixed.
2. Season with pepper according to your taste.
3. Serve and enjoy!

Nutrition (Per Serving)

- Calories: 358
- Fat: 30g
- Carbohydrates: 9g
- Protein: 14g

The Rutabaga Wedge Dish

Serving: 4
Prep Time: 15 minutes
Cook Time: 45 minutes
Ingredients:

- 2 medium rutabagas, medium, cleaned and peeled
- 4 tablespoons almond butter
- ½ teaspoon sunflower seeds
- ½ teaspoon onion powder
- 1/8 teaspoon black pepper
- ½ cup buffalo wing sauce
- ¼ cup blue cheese dressing, low fat and low sodium
- 2 green onions, chopped

How To:

1. Pre-heat your oven to 400 degrees F.
2. Line a baking sheet with parchment paper.
3. Wash and peel rutabagas, clean and peel them, and cut into wedge shapes.
4. Take a skillet and place it over low heat, add almond butter and melt.
5. Stir in onion powder, sunflower seeds, onion, black pepper.
6. Use seasoned almond butter to coat wedges.
7. Arrange wedges in a single layer on the baking sheet.
8. Bake for 30 minutes.
9. Remove and coat in buffalo sauce and return to oven.
10. Bake for 15 minutes more.
11. Place wedges on serving plate and trickle with blue cheese dressing.
12. Garnish with chopped green onion and enjoy!

Nutrition (Per Serving)

- Calories: 235
- Fat: 15g
- Carbohydrates: 10g
- Protein: 2.5g

Red Coleslaw

Serving: 4
Prep Time: 10 minutes
Cook Time: 0 minutes
Ingredients:

- 1 2/3 pounds red cabbage
- 2 tablespoons ground caraway seeds
- 1 tablespoon whole grain mustard
- 1 1/4 cups mayonnaise
- Sunflower seeds and black pepper

How To:

1. Take a large bowl and all the remaining ingredients.
2. Mix it well and let it sit for 10 minutes.
3. Serve and enjoy!

Nutrition (Per Serving)

- Calories: 406
- Fat: 40.8g
- Carbohydrates: 10g
- Protein: 2.2g

Classic Tuna Salad

Serving: 4
Prep Time: 10 minutes
Cook Time: Nil
SmartPoints: 1
Ingredients:

- 12 ounces white tuna, in water
- ½ cup celery, diced
- 2 tablespoons fresh parsley, chopped
- 2 tablespoons low-calorie mayonnaise, low fat and low sodium
- ½ teaspoon Dijon mustard
- ½ teaspoon sunflower seeds
- ¼ teaspoon fresh ground black pepper

Direction

1. Take a medium sized bowl and add tuna, parsley, and celery.
2. Mix well and add mayonnaise and mustard.
3. Season with pepper and sunflower seeds.
4. Stir and add olives, relish, chopped pickle, onion and mix well.
5. Serve and enjoy

Nutrition (Per Serving)

- Calories: 137
- Fat: 5g
- Carbohydrates: 1g
- Protein: 20g

Greek Salad

Serving: 4
Prep Time: 6 minutes
Cook Time: Nil
Ingredients:

- 2 cucumbers, diced
- 2 tomatoes, sliced
- 1 green lettuce, cut into thin strips
- 2 red bell peppers, cut
- ½ cup black olives pitted
- 3 ½ ounces feta cheese, cut
- 1 red onion, sliced
- 2 tablespoons olive oil
- 2 tablespoons lemon juice
- Sunflower seeds and pepper to taste

Direction

1. Dice cucumbers and slice up the tomatoes.
2. Tear the lettuce and cut it into thin strips.
3. De-seed and cut the peppers into strips.
4. Take a salad bowl and mix in all the listed vegetables, add olives and feta cheese (cut into cubes).
5. Take a small cup and mix in olive oil and lemon juice, season with sunflower seeds and pepper.
6. Pour mixture into the salad and toss well, enjoy!

Nutrition (Per Serving)

- Calories: 132
- Fat: 4g
- Carbohydrates: 3g
- Protein: 5g

Fancy Greek Orzo Salad

Serving: 4
Prep Time: 5 minutes and 24 hours chill time
Cook Time: 10 minutes
Ingredients:

- 1 cup orzo pasta, uncooked
- ½ cup fresh parsley, minced
- 6 teaspoons olive oil
- 1 onion, chopped
- 1 ½ teaspoons oregano

How To:

1. Cook the orzo and drain them.
2. Add to a serving dish.
3. Add 2 teaspoons of oil.
4. Take another dish and add parsley, onion, remaining oil and oregano.
5. Season with sunflower seeds, pepper according to your taste.
6. Pour the mixture over the orzo and let it chill for 24 hours.
7. Serve and enjoy at lunch!

Nutrition (Per Serving)

- Calories: 399
- Fat: 12g
- Carbohydrates: 55g
- Protein:16g

Homely Tuscan Tuna Salad

Serving: 4
Prep Time: 5-10 minutes
Cook Time: Nil
Ingredients:

- 15 ounces small white beans
- 6 ounces drained chunks of light tuna
- 10 cherry tomatoes, quartered
- 4 scallions, trimmed and sliced
- 2 tablespoons lemon juice

How To:

1. Add all of the listed ingredients to a bowl and gently stir.
2. Season with sunflower seeds and pepper accordingly, enjoy!

Nutrition (Per Serving)

- Calories: 322
- Fat: 8g
- Carbohydrates: 32g
- Protein:30g

Asparagus Loaded Lobster Salad

Serving: 4
Prep Time: 10 minutes
Cook Time: Nil
Smart Points: 5
Ingredients:

- 8 ounces lobster, cooked and chopped
- 3 ½ cups asparagus, chopped and steamed
- 2 tablespoons lemon juice
- 4 teaspoons extra virgin olive oil
- ¼ teaspoon kosher sunflower seeds
- Pepper
- ½ cup cherry tomatoes halved
- 1 basil leaf, chopped
- 2 tablespoons red onion, diced

How To:

1. Whisk in lemon juice, sunflower seeds, pepper in a bowl and mix with oil.
2. Take a bowl and add the rest of the ingredients.
3. Toss well and pour dressing on top.
4. Serve and enjoy!

Nutrition (Per Serving)

- Calories: 247
- Fat: 10g
- Carbohydrates: 14g
- Protein: 27g

Tasty Yogurt and Cucumber Salad

Serving: 4
Prep Time: 10 minutes
Cook Time: Nil
Ingredients:

- 5-6 small cucumbers, peeled and diced
- 1 (8 ounces) container plain Greek yogurt
- 2 garlic cloves, minced
- 1 tablespoon fresh mint, minced
- Sea sunflower seeds and fresh black pepper

How To:

1. Take a large bowl and add cucumbers, garlic, yogurt, mint.
2. Season with sunflower seeds and pepper.
3. Refrigerate the salad for 1 hour and serve.
4. Enjoy!

Nutrition (Per Serving)

- Calories: 74
- Fat: 0.7g
- Carbohydrates: 16g
- Protein: 2g

Unique Eggplant Salad

Serving: 3
Prep Time: 10 minutes
Cook Time: 30 minutes
Ingredients:

- 2 eggplants, peeled and sliced
- 2 garlic cloves
- 2 green bell pepper, sliced, seeds removed
- ½ cup fresh parsley
- ½ cup mayonnaise, low fat, low sodium
- Sunflower seeds and black pepper

How To:

1. Preheat your oven to 480 degrees F.
2. Take a baking pan and add eggplant, bell peppers and season with black pepper to it.
3. Bake for about 30 minutes.
4. Flip the vegetables after 20 minutes.
5. Then, take a bowl, add baked vegetables and all the remaining ingredients.
6. Mix well.
7. Serve and enjoy!

Nutrition (Per Serving)

- Calories: 196
- Fat: 108.g
- Carbohydrates: 13.4g
- Protein: 14.6g

Zucchini Pesto Salad

Serving: 4
Prep Time: 10 minutes
Cook Time: 10 minutes
Ingredients:

- 2 cups spiral pasta
- 2 zucchini, sliced and halved
- 4 tomatoes, cut
- 1 cup white mushrooms, cut
- 1 small red onion, chopped
- 2 tablespoons fresh basil leaves, chopped
- 2 tablespoons sunflower oil
- 1 tablespoon lemon juice
- Pepper and sunflower seeds to taste

How To:

1. Cook the pasta according to the package instructions, drain and rinse under cold water.
2. Take a large bowl and add zucchini, tomatoes, mushrooms, onion, and pasta.
3. Mix well,
4. In a food processor, add oil, lemon juice, basil, blue cheese, black, and process well.
5. Pour the mixture over the salad and toss well.
6. Serve and enjoy!

Nutrition (Per Serving)

- Calories: 301
- Fat: 25g
- Net Carbohydrates: 7g
- Protein: 10g

Wholesome Potato and Tuna Salad

Serving: 4
Prep Time: 10 minutes
Cook Time: nil
Ingredients:

- 1 pound baby potatoes, scrubbed, boiled
- 1 cup tuna chunks, drained
- 1 cup cherry tomatoes, halved
- 1 cup medium onion, thinly sliced
- 8 pitted black olives
- 2 medium hard-boiled eggs, sliced
- 1 head Romaine lettuce
- ¼ cup olive oil
- 2 tablespoons lemon juice
- 1 tablespoon Dijon mustard
- 1 teaspoon dill weed, chopped
- Pepper as needed

How To:

1. Take a small glass bowl and mix in your olive oil, lemon juice, Dijon mustard and dill.
2. Season the mix with pepper and salt.
3. Add in the tuna, baby potatoes, cherry tomatoes, red onion, green beans, black olives and toss everything nicely.
4. Arrange your lettuce leaves on a beautiful serving dish to make the base of your salad.
5. Top them with your salad mixture and place the egg slices.
6. Drizzle with the previously prepared Salad Dressing.
7. Serve hot

Nutrition (Per Serving)

- Calories: 406
- Fat: 22g
- Carbohydrates: 28g
- Protein: 26g

Baby Spinach Salad

Serving: 2
Prep Time: 10 minutes
Cook Time: nil
Ingredients:

- 1 bag baby spinach, washed and dried
- 1 red bell pepper, cut in slices
- 1 cup cherry tomatoes, cut in halves
- 1 small red onion, finely chopped
- 1 cup black olives, pitted

For dressing:

- 1 teaspoon dried oregano
- 1 large garlic clove
- 3 tablespoons red wine vinegar
- 4 tablespoons olive oil
- Sunflower seeds and pepper to taste

How To:

1. Prepare the dressing by blending in garlic, olive oil, vinegar in a food processor.
2. Take a large salad bowl and add spinach leaves, toss well with the dressing.
3. Add remaining ingredients and toss again, season with sunflower seeds and pepper and enjoy!

Nutrition (Per Serving)

- Calories: 126
- Fat: 10g
- Carbohydrates: 10g
- Protein: 2g

Elegant Corn Salad

Serving: 6
Prep Time: 10 minutes
Cooking Time: 2 hours
Ingredients:

- 2 ounces prosciutto, cut into strips
- 1 teaspoon olive oil
- 2 cups corn
- 1/2 cup salt-free tomato sauce
- 1 teaspoon garlic, minced
- 1 green bell pepper, chopped

How To:

1. Grease your Slow Cooker with oil.
2. Add corn, prosciutto, garlic, tomato sauce, bell pepper to your Slow Cooker.
3. Stir and place lid.
4. Cook on HIGH for 2 hours.
5. Divide between serving platters and enjoy!

Nutrition (Per Serving)

- Calories: 109
- Fat: 2g
- Carbohydrates: 10g
- Protein: 5g

Arabic Fattoush Salad

Serving: 4
Prep Time: 15 minutes
Cook Time: 2-3 minutes
Ingredients:

- 1 whole wheat pita bread
- 1 large English cucumber, diced
- 2 cup grape tomatoes, halved
- ½ medium red onion, finely diced
- ¾ cup fresh parsley, chopped
- ¾ cup mint leaves, chopped
- 1 clove garlic, minced
- ¼ cup fat free feta cheese, crumbled
- 1 tablespoon olive oil
- 1 teaspoon ground sumac
- Juice from ½ a lemon
- Salt and pepper as needed

How To:

1. Mist pita bread with cooking spray.
2. Season with salt.
3. Toast until the breads are crispy.
4. Take a large bowl and add the remaining ingredients and mix (except feta).
5. Top the mix with diced toasted pita and feta.
6. Serve and enjoy!

Nutrition (Per Serving)

- Calories: 86
- Fat: 3g
- Carbohydrates: 9g
- Protein: 9g

Heart Warming Cauliflower Salad

Serving: 3
Prep Time: 8 minutes
Cook Time: nil
Ingredients:

- 1 head cauliflower, broken into florets
- 1 small onion, chopped
- 1/8 cup extra virgin olive oil
- ¼ cup apple cider vinegar
- ½ teaspoon of sea salt
- ½ teaspoon of black pepper
- ¼ cup dried cranberries
- ¼ cup pumpkin seeds

How To:

1. Wash the cauliflower and break it up into small florets.
2. Transfer to a bowl.
3. Whisk oil, vinegar, salt and pepper in another bowl.
4. Add pumpkin seeds, cranberries to the bowl with dressing.
5. Mix well and pour the dressing over the cauliflower.
6. Add onions and toss.
7. Chill and serve.
8. Enjoy!

Nutrition (Per Serving)

- Calories: 163
- Fat: 11g
- Carbohydrates: 16g
- Protein: 3g

Great Greek Sardine Salad

Serving: 2
Prep Time: 10 minutes
Cook Time: 10 minutes
Ingredients:

- 2 tablespoons extra virgin olive oil
- 1 garlic clove, minced
- 2 teaspoons dried oregano
- ½ teaspoon freshly ground pepper
- 3 medium tomatoes, cut into large sized chunks
- 1 can (15 ounces) rinsed chickpeas
- 1/3 cup feta cheese, crumbled
- ¼ cup red onion, sliced
- 2 tablespoons Kalamata olives, sliced
- 2 cans 4 ounce drained sardines, with bones and packed in either oil or water

How To:

1. Take a large bowl and whisk in lemon juice, oregano, garlic, oil, pepper and mix well.
2. Add tomatoes, chickpeas, cucumber, olives, feta and mix.
3. Divide the salad amongst serving platter and top with sardines.
4. Enjoy!

Nutrition (Per Serving)

- Calories: 347
- Fat: 18g
- Carbohydrates: 29g
- Protein: 17g

Shrimp and Egg Medley

Serving: 4
Prep Time: 15 minutes
Cook Time: nil
Ingredients:

- 4 hard boiled eggs, peeled and chopped
- 1 pound cooked shrimp, peeled and deveined, chopped
- 1 sprig fresh dill, chopped
- ¼ cup mayonnaise
- 1 teaspoon Dijon mustard
- 4 fresh lettuce leaves

How To:

1. Take a large serving bowl and add the listed ingredients (except lettuce).
2. Stir well.
3. Serve over bed of lettuce leaves.
4. Enjoy!

Nutrition (Per Serving)

- Calories: 292
- Fat: 17g
- Carbohydrates: 1.6g
- Protein: 30g

Creamy Shrimp Salad

Serving: 4
Prep Time: 20 minutes
Cook Time: 5 minutes
Ingredients:

- 4 pounds large shrimp
- 1 lemon, quartered
- 3 cups celery stalks, chopped
- 1 red onion, chopped
- 2 cups mayonnaise
- 2 tablespoons white wine vinegar
- 1 teaspoon Dijon mustard
- Salt and pepper as needed

How To:

1. Take a large pan and place it over medium heat.
2. Add water (salted) and bring water to boil.
3. Add shrimp and lemon, cook for 3 minutes.
4. Let them cool.
5. Peel and de-vein the shrimps.
6. Take a large bowl and add cooked shrimp alongside remaining ingredients.
7. Stir well.
8. Serve immediately or chilled!

Nutrition (Per Serving)

- Calories: 153
- Fat: 5g
- Carbohydrates: 8g
- Protein: 19g

Passionate Quinoa and Black Bean Salad

Serving: 6
Prep Time: 5 minutes
Cook Time: 15 minutes
Ingredients:

- 1 cup uncooked quinoa
- 1 can 15 ounce black beans, drained and rinsed
- 1/3 cup cilantro, chopped
- 1 tablespoon olive oil
- 1 clove garlic, minced
- Juice from 1 lime
- Salt and pepper as needed

How To:

1. Cook quinoa according to the package instructions.
2. Transfer quinoa to a medium bowl and let it cool for 10 minutes.
3. Add remaining ingredients and toss well.
4. Serve and enjoy!

Nutrition (Per Serving)

- Calories: 188
- Fat: 4g
- Carbohydrates: 29g
- Protein: 8g

Zucchini Noodle Salad

Serving: 3
Prep Time: 15 minutes
Cook Time: nil
Ingredients:

- 2 large zucchini, spiralized/peeled into thin strips
- 1 small tomato, diced
- ¼ red onion, sliced thinly
- 1 large avocado, diced
- ½ cup olive oil
- ¼ cup balsamic vinegar
- 1 garlic clove, minced
- 2 teaspoons Dijon mustard
- Salt and pepper to taste
- ¼ cup blue cheese, crumbles

How To:

1. Take a large bowl and add zucchini noodles, onion, tomato, avocado.
2. Take a small bowl and whisk in olive oil, vinegar, mustard, garlic, salt and pepper.
3. Drizzle over salad and toss.
4. Divide into serving bowls and top with blue cheese crumbles.
5. Enjoy!

Nutrition (Per Serving)

- Calories: 770
- Fat: 74g
- Carbohydrates: 12g
- Protein: 8g

Onion and Orange Healthy Salad

Serving: 3
Prep Time: 10 minutes
Cook Time: nil
Ingredients:

- 6 large oranges
- 3 tablespoons red wine vinegar
- 6 tablespoons olive oil
- 1 teaspoon dried oregano
- 1 red onion, thinly sliced
- 1 cup olive oil
- ¼ cup fresh chives, chopped
- Ground black pepper

How To:

1. Peel the oranges and cut each of them in 4-5 crosswise slices.
2. Transfer the oranges to a shallow dish.
3. Drizzle vinegar, olive oil and sprinkle oregano.
4. Toss.
5. Chill for 30 minutes.
6. Arrange sliced onion and black olives on top.
7. Decorate with additional sprinkle of chives and fresh grind of pepper.
8. Serve and enjoy!

Nutrition (Per Serving)

- Calories: 120
- Fat: 6g
- Carbohydrates: 20g
- Protein: 2g

Stir Fried Almond and Spinach

Serving: 2
Prep Time: 10 minutes
Cook Time: 15 minutes
Ingredients:

- 34 pounds spinach
- 3 tablespoons almonds
- Salt to taste
- 1 tablespoon coconut oil

How To:

1. Add oil to a large pot and place on high heat.
2. Add spinach and let it cook, stirring frequently.
3. Once the spinach is cooked and tender, season with salt and stir.
4. Add almonds and enjoy!

Nutrition (Per Serving)

- Calories: 150
- Fat: 12g
- Carbohydrates: 10g
- Protein: 8g

Cilantro and Avocado Platter

Serving: 6
Prep Time: 10 minutes
Cook Time: nil
Ingredients:

- 2 avocados, peeled , pitted and diced
- 1 sweet onion, chopped
- 1 green bell pepper, chopped
- 1 large ripe tomato, chopped
- ¼ cup fresh cilantro, chopped
- ½ lime, juiced
- Salt and pepper as needed

How To:

1. Take a medium sized owl and add onion, bell pepper, tomato, avocados, lime and cilantro.
2. Mix well and give it a toss.
3. Season with salt and pepper according to your taste.
4. Serve and enjoy!

Nutrition (Per Serving)

- Calories: 126
- Fat: 10g
- Carbohydrates: 10g
- Protein: 2g

Chicken Breast Salad

Serving: 4
Prep Time: 25 minutes
Cook Time: 30-55 minutes
Ingredients:

- 3 ½ ounces chicken breast
- 2 tablespoons spinach
- 1 ¾ ounces lettuces
- 1 bell pepper
- 2 tablespoons olive oil
- Lemon juice to taste

How To:

1. Boil chicken breast without adding salt, cut the meat into small strips.
2. Put the spinach in boiling water for a few minute, cut into small strips .
3. Cut pepper in strips as well.
4. Add everything to a bowl and mix with juice and oil.
5. Serve!

Nutrition (Per Serving)

- Calories: 100
- Fat: 11g
- Carbohydrates: 3g
- Protein: 6g

Broccoli Salad

Serving: 1
Prep Time: 5 minutes
Cook Time: 10 minutes
Ingredients:

- 10 broccoli florets
- 2 red onions, sliced
- 1 ounce bacon, chopped into small pieces
- 1 cup coconut cream
- 1 teaspoon sesame seeds
- Salt

How To:

1. Cook bacon in hot oil until crispy.
2. Cook onions in fat left from the bacon.
3. Take a pan of boiling water and add broccoli florets, boil for a few minutes.
4. Take a salad bowl and add bacon pieces, onions, broccoli florets, coconut cream and salt.
5. Toss well and top with sesame seeds.
6. Enjoy!

Nutrition (Per Serving)

- Calories: 280
- Fat: 26g
- Carbohydrates: 8g
- Protein: 10g

Hearty Quinoa and Fruit Salad

Serving: 5
Prep Time: 5 minutes
Cook Time: 10 minutes
Ingredients:

- 3 ½ ounces Quinoa
- 3 peaches, diced
- 1 ½ ounces toasted hazelnuts, chopped
- Handful of mint, chopped
- Handful of parsley, chopped
- 2 tablespoons olive oil
- Zest of 1 lemon
- Juice of 1 lemon

How To:

1. Take medium sized saucepan and add quinoa.
2. Add 1 ¼ cups of water and bring it to a boil over medium-high heat.
3. Reduce the heat to low and simmer for 20 minutes.
4. Drain any excess liquid.
5. Add fruits, herbs, hazelnuts to the quinoa.
6. Allow it to cool and season.
7. Take a bowl and add olive oil, lemon zest and lemon juice.
8. Pour the mixture over the salad and give it a mix.
9. Enjoy!

Nutrition (Per Serving)

- Calories: 148
- Fat: 8g
- Carbohydrates: 16g
- Protein: 5g

Amazing Quinoa and Black Bean Salad

Serving: 4
Prep Time: 5 minutes
Cook Time: 2-3 minutes
Ingredients:

- 1 cup uncooked quinoa
- 1 can 15 ounce black beans, drained and rinsed
- 1/3 cup cilantro, chopped
- 1 tablespoon olive oil
- 1 clove garlic, minced
- Juice from 1 lime
- Salt and pepper as needed

How To:

1. Cook quinoa according to package instructions.
2. Transfer quinoa to a medium bowl and allow it to cool for 10 minutes.
3. Add the rest of the ingredients and toss.
4. Serve and enjoy!
5. Enjoy!

Nutrition (Per Serving)

- Calories: 188
- Fat: 4g
- Carbohydrates: 29g
- Protein: 8g

Authentic Mediterranean Pearl and Couscous

Serving: 4
Prep Time: 15 minutes
Cook Time: 10 minutes l
Ingredients:
For The Vinaigrette

- 1 large lemon, juiced
- 1/3 cup extra virgin olive oil
- 1 teaspoon dill weed
- 1 teaspoon garlic powder
- Salt and pepper as needed

For Israeli Couscous

- 2 cups Pearl Couscous
- Extra virgin olive oil
- 2 cups grape tomatoes, halved
- Water as needed
- 1/3 cup red onions, chopped
- ½ English Cucumber, chopped
- 15 ounces chickpeas
- 14 ounce (can) fresh artichoke hearts, chopped
- ½ cup kalamata olives, pitted
- 15-20 pieces fresh basil leaves, torn and chopped
- 3 ounces fresh baby mozarella cheese

How To:

1. Start by preparing the vinaigrette. Take a bowl and add the ingredients listed under vinaigrette.
2. Mix them well and keep it on the side.
3. Take a medium sized heavy pot and place it over medium heat.
4. Add 2 tablespoons of olive oil and allow it to heat up.
5. Add couscous and keep cooking until golden brown.
6. Add 3 cups of boiling water and cook the couscous according to package instructions.
7. Once done, drain in a colander and keep on the side.
8. Take another large sized mixing bowl and add the rest of the ingredients, except cheese and basil.

9. Add the cooked couscous and basil to the mix and mix everything well.
10. Give the vinaigrette a nice stir and whisk it into the couscous salad.
11. Mix well.
12. Adjust the seasoning as required.
13. Add mozzarella cheese.
14. Garnish with some basil.
15. Enjoy!

Nutrition (Per Serving)

- Calories: 393
- Fat: 13g
- Carbohydrates: 57g
- Protein: 13g

Mesmerizing Fruit Bowl

Serving: 1
Prep Time: 30 minutes
Cook Time: nil
Ingredients:

- 2 fresh ripe mangoes
- 2 cups pineapple chunks
- Fresh pineapple tips
- 1 banana, sliced
- 1-2 cups fresh papaya, cubed
- 1 kiwi fruit, cubed
- 2 cups seedless grapes, halved
- ¼ cup coconut milk
- 2 tablespoons lime juice
- 3-4 tablespoons sugar
- Strawberries, cranberries or raspberries as topping

How To:

1. Slice the fruits above, except the contrasting red ones such as dried cranberries, raspberries and strawberries.
2. Add them to your mixing bowl and drizzle a bit of lime juice on top.
3. Stir well and sprinkle a bit of sugar on top, give it a nice stir.
4. Allow it to chill for 30 minutes and serve the salad with a bit of coconut milk.
5. Season the sweetness accordingly and top it with some cranberries, raspberries and strawberries.
6. Enjoy!

Nutrition (Per Serving)

- Calories: 209
- Fat: 0g
- Carbohydrates: 43g
- Protein: 2g

Tangy Strawberry Salad

Serving: 4
Prep Time: 15 minutes
Cook Time: nil
Ingredients:

- 4 slices bacon, cooked and crumbled
- 10 large strawberries, stem removed and sliced
- 4 cups baby spinach
- 1 avocado, chopped

For Dressing

- Zest of 1 lemon
- ¼ red onion, minced
- ¼ cup red wine vinegar
- 1 tablespoon Dijon mustard
- 1 lemon, juiced
- 1 teaspoon poppy seed
- ½ cup extra light olive oil

How To:

1. Add all the dressing ingredients to a blender and blend until you have a smooth mixture (except poppy seeds).
2. Stir in poppy seeds after blending.
3. Take a large bowl and toss strawberries, bacon, spinach and avocado.
4. Mix well and drizzle the dressing on top.
5. Serve and enjoy!

Nutrition (Per Serving)

- Calories: 96
- Fat: 1g
- Carbohydrates: 22g
- Protein: 3g

Peachful Applesauce Salad

Serving: 6
Prep Time: 15 minutes
Cook Time: nil
Ingredients:

- 1 cup diet lemon lime-soda
- 1 pack sugar-free fruit mixed peach gelatin
- 1 cup unsweetened applesauce
- 2 cups coconut whip cream
- 1/8 teaspoon ground nutmeg
- 1/8 teaspoon vanilla extract
- 1 fresh peach, peeled and chopped

How To:

1. Take a saucepan and bring the soda to a boil over medium heat.
2. Remove heat.
3. Stir in sugar-free peach gelatin until dissolved.
4. Add applesauce and stir.
5. Let it chill until partially set.
6. Fold in whipped topping and vanilla extract.
7. Fold in the peach and wait until firm.
8. Serve and enjoy!

Nutrition (Per Serving)

- Calories: 354
- Fat: 17g
- Carbohydrates: 37g
- Protein: 15g

The Citrus Lover's Salad

Serving: 16
Prep Time: 10 minutes
Cook Time: nil
Ingredients:

- 1 medium zucchini, julienned
- ½ cup olive oil
- 1 medium red onion, sliced
- 1 cup fresh broccoli, cut into florets
- 1 cup fresh cauliflower florets
- 1/8 teaspoon pepper
- 1 medium cucumber, halved and sliced
- ¼ cup white wine vinegar
- 1 teaspoon dried oregano
- 1 medium carrot, julienned
- ½ teaspoon ground mustard
- ¼ teaspoon garlic powder
- 1/8 teaspoon celery salt

How To:

1. Add olives and veggies to a small bowl.
2. Take another bowl and whisk in vinegar, seasoning, oil.
3. Pour the mixture over veggies and toss.
4. Let sit for 3 hours.
5. Serve and enjoy!

Nutrition (Per Serving)

- Calories: 72
- Fat: 7g
- Carbohydrates: 2g
- Protein: 2g

Wicked Vanilla Fruit Salad

Serving: 5
Prep Time: 10 minutes
Cook Time: nil
Ingredients:

- 8 cans mandarin orange, drained
- 4 packs instant vanilla pudding mix
- 6 cans pineapple chunks
- 10 medium red apples, chopped

How To:

1. Drain pineapples, making sure to reserve the liquid.
2. Keep them on the side.
3. Add cold water to the juice to make 6 cups liquid in total.
4. Whisk the juice mix and pudding mix into a large bowl for about 2 minutes.
5. Let it stand for 2 minutes until soft-set.
6. Stir in apples, oranges and reserved pineapple.
7. Chill in fridge and serve.
8. Enjoy!

Nutrition (Per Serving)

- Calories: 33
- Fat: 0g
- Carbohydrates: 8g
- Protein: 0g

Green Papaya Salad

Serving: 6
Prep Time: 10 minutes
Cook Time: nil
Ingredients:

- 10 small shrimps, dried
- 2 small red Thai Chilies
- 1 garlic clove, peeled
- ¼ cup tamarind juice
- 1 tablespoon palm sugar
- 1 tablespoon Thai fish sauce, low sodium
- 1 lime, cut into 1-inch pieces
- 4 cherry tomatoes, halved
- 3 long beans, trimmed into 1-inch pieces
- 1 carrot, coarsely shredded
- ½ English cucumber, coarsely chopped and seeded
- 1/6 small green cabbage, cored and thinly sliced
- 1 pound unripe green papaya, quartered, seeded and shredded using a mandolin
- 3 tablespoons unsalted roasted peanuts

How To:

1. Take a mortar and pestle and crush your shrimp alongside garlic, chilies.
2. Add tamarind juice, fish sauce and palm sugar.
3. Squeeze the juice from the lime pieces and pour 3 quarts over the mortar.
4. Grind the mixture in the mortar to make a dressing, keep the dressing on the side.
5. Take a bowl, add the remaining ingredients (excluding the peanut), making sure to add the papaya last.
6. Use a spoon and stir in the dressing.
7. Mix the vegetables and fruit and coat them well.
8. Transfer to your serving dish.
9. Garnish with some peanuts and lime pieces.
10. Enjoy!

Nutrition (Per Serving)

- Calories: 316
- Fat: 13g
-
- Carbohydrates: 5g
- Protein: 11g

Pineapple, Papaya and Mango Delight

Serving: 2
Prep Time: 20 minutes
Cook Time: nil
Ingredients:

- 1 pound fresh pineapple, peeled and cut into chunks
- 1 mango, peeled, pitted and cubed
- 2 papayas, peeled, seeded and cubed
- 3 tablespoons fresh lime juice
- ¼ cup fresh mint leaves, chopped

How To:

1. Take a large bowl and add the listed ingredients.
2. Toss well to coat.
3. Put in fridge and chill.
4. Serve and enjoy!

Nutrition (Per Serving)

- Calories: 292
- Fat: 11g
- Carbohydrates: 42g
- Protein: 8g

Cashew and Green Apple Salad

Serving: 2
Prep Time: 15 minutes
Cook Time: nil
Ingredients:

- ½ large apple, cored and sliced
- 2 cups mixed fresh greens
- 1 tablespoon unsalted cashews
- 1 tablespoon apple cider vinegar

How To:

1. Take a serving bowl and add apple, cashews and greens.
2. Drizzle apple cider vinegar on top.
3. Serve immediately!

Nutrition (Per Serving)

- Calories: 118
- Fat: 4g
- Carbohydrates: 19g
- Protein: 3g

Watermelon and Tomato Mix

Serving: 2
Prep Time: 20 minutes
Cook Time: nil
Ingredients:

- 1 large red tomato, cubed
- 1 large yellow tomato, cubed

Dressing

- ¼ cup olive oil
- ¼ cup rice wine vinegar
- 2 teaspoons honey
- 2 cups fresh watermelon, peeled, seeded and cubed

- 2 tablespoons chili garlic sauce
- 1 tablespoon fresh lemon basil, chopped
- Salt and pepper as needed

How To:

1. Take a large bowl and add all the salad ingredients.
2. Take another bowl and add the dressing ingredients.
3. Beat well until combined.
4. Pour dressing over salad and toss.
5. Serve and enjoy!

Nutrition (Per Serving)

- Calories: 87
- Fat: 7g
- Carbohydrates: 7g
- Protein: 0.6g

Chapter 10: Side Dish Recipes

Hearty Cashew and Almond Butter

Serving: 1 and ½ cups
Prep Time: 5 minutes
Cook Time: Nil
Ingredients:

- 1 cup almonds, blanched
- 1/3 cup cashew nuts
- 2 tablespoons coconut oil
- ½ teaspoon cinnamon

How To:

1. Pre-heat your oven to 350 degrees F.
2. Bake almonds and cashews for 12 minutes.
3. Let them cool.
4. Transfer to food processor and add remaining ingredients.
5. Add oil and keep blending until smooth.
7. Serve and enjoy!

Nutrition (Per Serving)

- Calories: 205
- Fat: 19g
- Carbohydrates: g
- Protein: 2.8g

Red Coleslaw

Serving: 4
Prep Time: 10 minutes
Cook Time: 0 minutes
Ingredients:

- 1 2/3 pounds red cabbage
- 2 tablespoons ground caraway seeds
- 1 tablespoon whole grain mustard
- 1 1/4 cups mayonnaise, low fat, low sodium
- Salt and black pepper

How To:

1. Cut the red cabbage into small slices.
2. Take a large-sized bowl and add all the ingredients alongside cabbage.
3. Mix well, season with salt and pepper.
4. Serve and enjoy!

Nutrition (Per Serving)

- Calories: 406
- Fat: 40.8g
- Carbohydrates: 10g
- Protein: 2.2g

Avocado Mayo Medley

Serving: 4
Prep Time: 5 minutes
Cook Time: Nil
Ingredients:

- 1 medium avocado, cut into chunks
- ½ teaspoon ground cayenne pepper
- 2 tablespoons fresh cilantro
- ¼ cup olive oil
- ½ cup mayo, low fat and los sodium

How To:

1. Take a food processor and add avocado, cayenne pepper, lime juice, salt and cilantro.
2. Mix until smooth.
3. Slowly incorporate olive oil, add 1 tablespoon at a time and keep processing between additions.
4. Store and use as needed!

Nutrition (Per Serving)

- Calories: 231
- Fat: 20g
- Carbohydrates: 5g
- Protein: 3g

Amazing Garlic Aioli

Serving: 4
Prep Time: 5 minutes
Cook Time: Nil
Ingredients:

- ½ cup mayonnaise, low fat and low sodium
- 2 garlic cloves, minced
- Juice of 1 lemon
- 1 tablespoon fresh-flat leaf Italian parsley, chopped
- 1 teaspoon chives, chopped
- Salt and pepper to taste

How To:

1. Add mayonnaise, garlic, parsley, lemon juice, chives and season with salt and pepper.
2. Blend until combined well.
3. Pour into refrigerator and chill for 30 minutes.
4. Serve and use as needed!

Nutrition (Per Serving)

- Calories: 813
- Fat: 88g
- Carbohydrates: 9g
- Protein: 2g

Easy Seed Crackers

Serving: 72 crackers
Prep Time: 10 minutes
Cooking Time: 60 minutes
Ingredients:

- 1 cup boiling water
- 1/3 cup chia seeds
- 1/3 cup sesame seeds
- 1/3 cup pumpkin seeds
- 1/3 cup Flaxseeds
- 1/3 cup sunflower seeds
- 1 tablespoon Psyllium powder
- 1 cup almond flour
- 1 teaspoon salt
- ¼ cup coconut oil, melted

How To:

1. Pre-heat your oven to 300 degrees F.
2. Line a cookie sheet with parchment paper and keep it on the side.
3. Add listed ingredients (except coconut oil and water) to food processor and pulse until ground.
4. Transfer to a large mixing bowl and pour melted coconut oil and boiling water, mix.
5. Transfer mix to prepared sheet and spread into a thin layer.
6. Cut dough into crackers and bake for 60 minutes.
7. Cool and serve.
8. Enjoy!

Nutrition (Per Serving)

- Total Carbs: 10.6g
- Fiber: 3g
- Protein: 5g
- Fat: 14.6g

Hearty Almond Crackers

Serving: 40 crackers
Prep Time: 10 minutes
Cooking Time: 20 minutes
Ingredients:

- 1 cup almond flour
- ¼ teaspoon baking soda
- 1/8 teaspoon black pepper
- 3 tablespoons sesame seeds
- 1 egg, beaten
- Salt and pepper to taste

How To:

1. Pre-heat your oven to 350 degrees F.
2. Line two baking sheets with parchment paper and keep them on the side.
3. Mix the dry ingredients in a large bowl and add egg, mix well and form dough.
4. Divide dough into two balls.
5. Roll out the dough between two pieces of parchment paper.
6. Cut into crackers and transfer them to prepared baking sheet.
7. Bake for 15-20 minutes.
8. Repeat until all the dough has been used up.
9. Leave crackers to cool and serve.
10. Enjoy!

Nutrition (Per Serving)

- Total Carbs: 8g
- Fiber: 2g
- Protein: 9g
- Fat: 28g

Black Bean Salsa

Serving: 4
Prep Time: 10 minutes
Cook Time: Nil
Ingredients:

- 1 tablespoon coconut aminos
- ½ teaspoon cumin, ground
- 1 cup canned black beans, no salt
- 1 cup salsa
- 6 cups romaine lettuce, torn
- ½ cup avocado, peeled, pitted and cubed

How To:

1. Take a bowl and add beans, alongside other ingredients.
2. Toss well and serve.
3. Enjoy!

Nutrition (Per Serving)

- Calories: 181
- Fat: 5g
- Carbohydrates: 14g
- Protein: 7g

Corn Spread

Serving: 4
Prep Time: 10 minutes
Cook Time: 10 minutes
Ingredients:

- 30 ounce canned corn, drained
- 2 green onions, chopped
- ½ cup coconut cream
- 1 jalapeno, chopped
- ½ teaspoon chili powder

How To:

1. Take a pan and add corn, green onions, jalapeno, chili powder, stir well.
2. Bring to a simmer over medium heat and cook for 10 minutes.
3. Let it chill and add coconut cream.
4. Stir well.
5. Serve and enjoy!

Nutrition (Per Serving)

- Calories: 192
- Fat: 5g
- Carbohydrates: 11g
- Protein: 8g

Moroccan Leeks Snack

Serving: 4
Prep Time: 10 minutes
Cook Time: nil
Ingredients:

- 1 bunch radish, sliced
- 3 cups leeks, chopped
- 1 ½ cups olives, pitted and sliced
- Pinch turmeric powder
- 2 tablespoons essential olive oil
- 1 cup cilantro, chopped

How To:

1. Take a bowl and mix in radishes, leeks, olives and cilantro.
2. Mix well.
3. Season with pepper, oil, turmeric and toss well.
4. Serve and enjoy!

Nutrition (Per Serving)

- Calories: 120
- Fat: 1g
- Carbohydrates: 1g
- Protein: 6g

The Bell Pepper Fiesta

Serving: 4
Prep Time: 10 minutes
Cook Time: nil
Ingredients:

- 2 tablespoons dill, chopped
- 1 yellow onion, chopped
- 1 pound multi colored peppers, cut, halved, seeded and cut into thin strips
- 3 tablespoons organic olive oil
- 2 ½ tablespoons white wine vinegar
- Black pepper to taste

How To:

1. Take a bowl and mix in sweet pepper, onion, dill, pepper, oil, vinegar and toss well.
2. Divide between bowls and serve.
3. Enjoy!

Nutrition (Per Serving)

- Calories: 120
- Fat: 3g
- Carbohydrates: 1g
- Protein: 6g

Spiced Up Pumpkin Seeds Bowls

Serving: 4
Prep Time: 10 minutes
Cook Time: 20 minutes
Ingredients:

- ½ tablespoon chili powder
- ½ teaspoon cayenne
- 2 cups pumpkin seeds
- 2 teaspoons lime juice

How To:

1. Spread pumpkin seeds over lined baking sheet, add lime juice, cayenne and chili powder.
2. Toss well.
3. Pre-heat your oven to 275 degrees F.
4. Roast in your oven for 20 minutes and transfer to small bowls.
5. Serve and enjoy!

Nutrition (Per Serving)

- Calories: 170
- Fat: 3g
- Carbohydrates: 10g
- Protein: 6g

Mozzarella Cauliflower Bars

Serving: 4
Prep Time: 10 minutes
Cook Time: 40 minutes
Ingredients:

- 1 cauliflower head, riced
- 12 cup low-fat mozzarella cheese, shredded
- ¼ cup egg whites
- 1 teaspoon Italian dressing, low fat
- Pepper to taste

How To:

1. Spread cauliflower rice over lined baking sheet.
2. Pre-heat your oven to 375 degrees F.
3. Roast for 20 minutes.
4. Transfer to bowl and spread pepper, cheese, seasoning, egg whites and stir well.
5. Spread in a rectangular pan and press.
6. Transfer to oven and cook for 20 minutes more.
7. Serve and enjoy!

Nutrition (Per Serving)

- Calories: 140
- Fat: 2g
- Carbohydrates: 6g
- Protein: 6g

Tomato Pesto Crackers

Serving: 4
Prep Time: 10 minutes
Cook Time: 15 minutes
Ingredients:

- 1 ¼ cups almond flour
- ½ teaspoon garlic powder
- ½ teaspoon baking powder
- 2 tablespoons sun-dried tomato Pesto
- 3 tablespoons ghee
- ½ teaspoon dried basil
- ¼ teaspoon pepper

How To:

1. Pre-heat your oven to 325 degrees F.
2. Take a bowl and add listed ingredients.
3. Mix well and combine.
4. Take a baking sheet lined with parchment paper and spread the dough.
5. Transfer to oven and bake for 15 minutes.
6. Break into small sized crackers and serve.
7. Enjoy!

Nutrition (Per Serving)

- Calories: 204
- Fat: 20g
- Carbohydrates: 3g
- Protein: 3g

Garlic Cottage Cheese Crispy

Serving: 4
Prep Time: 5 minutes
Cook Time: 2 minutes
Ingredients:

- 1 cup cottage cheese
- ½ teaspoon Garlic powder
- Pinch of pepper
- Pinch of onion powder

How To:

1. Take a skillet and place it over medium heat.
2. Take a bowl and mix in cheese and spices.
3. Scoop half a teaspoon of the cheese mix and place in the pan.
4. Cook for 1 minute per side.
5. Repeat until done.
6. Enjoy!

Nutrition (Per Serving)

- Calories: 70
- Fat: 6g
- Carbohydrates: 1g
- Protein: 6g

Tasty Cucumber Bites

Serving: 4
Prep Time: 5 minutes
Cook Time: nil
Ingredients:

- 1 (8 ounce) cream cheese container, low fat
- 1 tablespoon bell pepper, diced
- 1 tablespoon shallots, diced
- 1 tablespoon parsley, chopped
- 2 cucumbers
- Pepper to taste

How To:

1. Take a bowl and add cream cheese, onion, pepper, parsley.
2. Peel cucumbers and cut in half.
3. Remove seeds and stuff with cheese mix.
4. Cut into bite sized portions and enjoy!

Nutrition (Per Serving)

- Calories: 85
- Fat: 4g
- Carbohydrates: 2g
- Protein: 3g

Juicy Simple Lemon Fat Bombs

Serving: 3
Prep Time: 10 minutes
Cooking Time: /
Freeze Time: 2 hours
Ingredients:

- 1 whole lemon
- 4 ounces cream cheese
- 2 ounces butter
- 2 teaspoons natural sweetener

How To:

1. Take a fine grater and zest your lemon.
2. Squeeze lemon juice into a bowl alongside the zest.
3. Add butter, cream cheese to a bowl and add zest, salt, sweetener and juice.
4. Stir well using a hand mixer until smooth.
5. Spoon mix into molds and freeze for 2 hours.
6. Serve and enjoy!

Nutrition (Per Serving)

- Total Carbs: 4g
- Fiber: 1g
- Protein: 4g
- Fat: 43g
- Calories: 404

Chocolate Coconut Bombs

Serving: 12
Prep Time: 20 minutes
Cooking Time: None
Freeze Time: 1 hour
Ingredients:

- ½ cup dark cocoa powder
- ½ tablespoon vanilla extract
- 5 drops stevia
- 1 cup coconut oil, solid
- 1 tablespoon peppermint extract

How To:

1. Take a high speed food processor and add all the ingredients.
2. Blend until combined.
3. Take a teaspoon and drop a spoonful onto parchment paper.
4. Refrigerate until solidified and keep refrigerated.

Nutrition (Per Serving)

- Total Carbs: 0g
- Fiber: 0g
- Protein: 0g
- Fat: 14g
- Calories: 126

Terrific Jalapeno Bacon Bombs

Serving: 2
Prep Time: 15 minutes
Cook Time: 10 minutes
Ingredients:

- 12 large jalapeno peppers
- 16 bacon strips
- 6 ounces full fat cream cheese
- 2 teaspoon garlic powder
- 1 teaspoon chili powder

How To:

1. Pre-heat your oven to 350 degrees F.
2. Place a wire rack over a roasting pan and keep it on the side.
3. Make a slit lengthways across jalapeno pepper and scrape out the seeds, discard them.
4. Place a nonstick skillet over high heat and add half of your bacon strips, cook until crispy.
5. Drain them.
6. Chop the cooked bacon strips and transfer to large bowl.
7. Add cream cheese and mix.
8. Season the cream cheese and bacon mix with garlic and chili powder.
9. Mix well.
10. Stuff the mix into the jalapeno peppers with and wrap a raw bacon strip all around.
11. Arrange the stuffed wrapped jalapeno on prepared wire rack.
12. Roast for 10 minutes.
13. Transfer to cooling rack and serve!

Nutrition (Per Serving)

- Calories: 209
- Fat: 9g
- Net Carbohydrates: 15g
- Protein: 9g

Yummy Espresso Fat Bombs

Serving: 24
Prep Time: 20 minutes
Cooking Time: nil
Freeze Time: 4 hours
Ingredients:

- 5 tablespoons butter, tender
- 3 ounces cream cheese, soft
- 2 ounces espresso
- 4 tablespoons coconut oil
- 2 tablespoons coconut whipping cream
- 2 tablespoons stevia

How To:

1. Prepare your double boiler and melt all ingredients (except stevia) for 3-4 minutes and mix.
2. Add sweetener and mix using hand mixer.
3. Spoon mixture into silicone muffin molds and freeze for 4 hours.
4. Remove fat bombs and enjoy!

Nutrition (Per Serving)

- Total Carbs: 1.3g
- Fiber: 0.2g
- Protein: 0.3g
- Fat: 7g

Crispy Coconut Bombs

Serving: 6
Prep Time: 10 minutes
Cooking Time: /
Freeze Time: 1-2 hours
Ingredients:

- 14 ½ ounces coconut milk
- ¾ cup coconut oil
- 1 cup unsweetened coconut flakes
- 20 drops stevia

How To:

1. Microwave your coconut oil for 20 seconds in microwave.
2. Mix in coconut milk and stevia in the hot oil.
3. Stir in coconut flakes and pour the mixture into molds.
4. Let it chill for 60 minutes in fridge.
5. Serve and enjoy!

Nutrition (Per Serving)

- Total Carbs: 2g
- Fiber: 0.5g
- Protein: 1g
- Fat: 13g
- Calories: 123
- Net Carbs: 1g

Pumpkin Pie Fat Bombs

Serving: 12
Prep Time: 35 minutes
Cooking Time: 5 minutes
Freeze Time: 3 hours
Ingredients:

- 2 tablespoons coconut oil
- 1/3 cup pumpkin puree
- 1/3 cup almond oil
- ¼ cup almond oil
- 3 ounces sugar-free dark chocolate
- 1 ½ teaspoons pumpkin pie spice mix
- Stevia to taste

How To:

1. Melt almond oil and dark chocolate over a double boiler.
2. Take this mixture and layer the bottom of 12 muffin cups.
3. Freeze until the crust has set.
4. Meanwhile, take a saucepan and combine the rest of the ingredients.
5. Put the saucepan on low heat.
6. Heat until softened and mix well.
7. Pour this over the initial chocolate mixture.
8. Let it chill for at least 1 hour.

Nutrition (Per Serving)

- Total Carbs: 3g
- Fiber: 1g
- Protein: 3g
- Fat: 13g
- Calories: 124

Sensational Lemonade Fat Bomb

Serving: 2
Prep Time: 2 hours
Cook Time: Nil
Ingredients:

- ½ lemon
- 4 ounces cream cheese
- 2 ounces almond butter
- Salt to taste
- 2 teaspoons natural sweetener

How To:

1. Take a fine grater and zest lemon.
2. Squeeze lemon juice into bowl with zest.
3. Add butter, cream cheese in a bowl and add zest, juice, salt, sweetener.
4. Mix well using a hand mixer until smooth.
5. Spoon mixture into molds and let them freeze for 2 hours.
6. Serve and enjoy!

Nutrition (Per Serving)

- Calories: 404
- Fat: 43g
- Carbohydrates: 4g
- Protein: 4g

Sweet Almond and Coconut Fat Bombs

Serving: 6
Prep Time: 10 minutes
Cooking Time: /
Freeze Time: 20 minutes
Ingredients:

- ¼ cup melted coconut oil
- 9 ½ tablespoons almond butter
- 90 drops liquid stevia
- 3 tablespoons cocoa
- 9 tablespoons melted butter, salted

How To:

1. Take a bowl and add all of the listed ingredients.
2. Mix them well.
3. Pour scant 2 tablespoons of the mixture into as many muffin molds as you like.
4. Chill for 20 minutes and pop them out.
5. Serve and enjoy!

Nutrition (Per Serving)

- Total Carbs: 2g
- Fiber: 0g
- Protein: 2.53g
- Fat: 14g

Almond and Tomato Balls

Serving: 6
Prep Time: 10 minutes
Cooking Time: /
Freeze Time: 20 minutes
Ingredients:

- 1/3 cup pistachios, de-shelled
- 10 ounces cream cheese
- 1/3 cup sun dried tomatoes, diced

How To:

1. Chop pistachios into small pieces.
2. Add cream cheese, tomatoes in a bowl and mix well.
3. Chill for 15-20 minutes and turn into balls.
4. Roll into pistachios.
5. Serve and enjoy!

Nutrition (Per Serving)

- Carb: 183
- Fat: 18g
- Carb: 5g
- Protein: 5g

Avocado Tuna Bites

Serving: 4
Prep Time: 10 minutes
Cook Time: nil
Ingredients:

- 1/3 cup coconut oil
- 1 avocado, cut into cubes
- 10 ounces canned tuna, drained
- ¼ cup parmesan cheese, grated
- ¼ teaspoon garlic powder
- 1/4 teaspoon onion powder
- 1/3 cup almond flour
- ¼ teaspoon pepper
- ¼ cup low fat mayonnaise
- Pepper as needed

How To:

1. Take a bowl and add tuna, mayo, flour, parmesan, spices and mix well.
2. Fold in avocado and make 12 balls out of the mixture.
3. Melt coconut oil in pan and cook over medium heat, until all sides are golden.
4. Serve and enjoy!

Nutrition (Per Serving)

- Calories: 185
- Fat: 18g
- Carbohydrates: 1g
- Protein: 5g

Mediterranean Pop Corn Bites

Serving: 4
Prep Time: 5 minutes + 20 minutes chill time
Cook Time: 2-3 minutes
Ingredients:

- 3 cups Medjool dates, chopped
- 12 ounces brewed coffee
- 1 cup pecan, chopped
- ½ cup coconut, shredded
- ½ cup cocoa powder

How To:

1. Soak dates in warm coffee for 5 minutes.
2. Remove dates from coffee and mash them, making a fine smooth mixture.
3. Stir in remaining ingredients (except cocoa powder) and form small balls out of the mixture.
4. Coat with cocoa powder, serve and enjoy!

Nutrition (Per Serving)

- Calories: 265
- Fat: 12g
- Carbohydrates: 43g
- Protein 3g

Hearty Buttery Walnuts

Serving: 4
Prep Time: 10 minutes
Cook Time: nil
Ingredients:

- 4 walnut halves
- ½ tablespoon almond butter

How To:
1. Spread butter over two walnut halves.
2. Top with other halves.
3. Serve and enjoy!

Nutrition (Per Serving)

- Calories: 90
- Fat: 10g
- Carbohydrates: 0g
- Protein: 1g

Refreshing Watermelon Sorbet

Serving: 4
Prep Time: 20 minutes + 20 hours chill time
Cook Time: Nil
Ingredients:

- 4 cups watermelon, seedless and chunked
- ¼ cup coconut sugar
- 2 tablespoons lime juice

How To:
1. Add the listed ingredients to a blender and puree.
2. Transfer to a freezer container with a tight-fitting lid.
3. Freeze the mix for about 4-6 hours until you have gelatin-like consistency.
4. Puree the mix once again in batches and return to the container.
5. Chill overnight.
6. Allow the sorbet to stand for 5 minutes before serving and enjoy!

Nutrition (Per Serving)

- Calories: 91
- Fat: 0g
- Carbohydrates: 25g
- Protein: 1g

Lovely Faux Mac and Cheese

Serving: 4
Prep Time: 15 minutes
Cook Time: 45 minutes
Ingredients:

- 5 cups cauliflower florets
- Salt and pepper to taste
- 1 cup coconut milk
- ½ cup vegetable broth
- 2 tablespoons coconut flour, sifted
- 1 organic egg, beaten
- 2 cups cheddar cheese

How To:

1. Pre-heat your oven to 350 degrees F.
2. Season florets with salt and steam until firm.
3. Place florets in greased ovenproof dish.
4. Heat coconut milk over medium heat in a skillet, make sure to season the oil with salt and pepper.
5. Stir in broth and add coconut flour to the mix, stir.
6. Cook until the sauce begins to bubble.
7. Remove heat and add beaten egg.
8. Pour the thick sauce over cauliflower and mix in cheese.
9. Bake for 30-45 minutes.
10. Serve and enjoy!

Nutrition (Per Serving)

- Calories: 229
- Fat: 14g
- Carbohydrates: 9g
- Protein: 15g

Beautiful Banana Custard

Serving: 3
Prep Time: 10 minutes
Cook Time: 25 minutes
Ingredients:

- 2 ripe bananas, peeled and mashed finely
- ½ teaspoon of vanilla extract
- 14-ounce unsweetened almond milk
- 3 eggs

How To:

1. Pre-heat your oven to 350 degrees F.
2. Grease 8 custard glasses lightly.
3. Arrange the glasses in a large baking dish.
4. Take a large bowl and mix all of the ingredients and mix them well until combined nicely.
5. Divide the mixture evenly between the glasses.
6. Pour water in the baking dish.
7. Bake for 25 minutes.
8. Take out and serve.
9. Enjoy!

Nutrition (Per Serving)

- Calories: 59
- Fat: 2.4g
- Carbohydrates: 7g
- Protein: 3g

Healthy Tahini Buns

Serving: 3 buns
Prep Time: 10 minutes
Cooking Time: 15-20 minutes
Ingredients:

- 1 whole egg
- 5 tablespoons Tahini paste
- ½ teaspoon baking soda
- 1 teaspoon lemon juice
- 1 pinch salt

How To:

1. Pre-heat your oven to 350 degrees F.
2. Line a baking sheet with parchment paper and keep it on the side.
3. Add the listed ingredients to a blender and blend until you have a smooth batter.
4. Scoop batter onto prepared sheet forming buns.
5. Bake for 15-20 minutes.
6. Once done, remove from oven and let them cool.
7. Serve and enjoy!

Nutrition (Per Serving)

- Total Carbs: 7g
- Fiber: 2g
- Protein: 6g
- Fat: 14g
- Calories: 172

Spicy Pecan Bowl

Serving: 3
Prep Time: 10 minutes
Cook Time: 120 minutes
Ingredients:

- 1 pound pecans, halved
- 2 tablespoons olive oil
- 1 teaspoon basil, dried
- 1 tablespoon chili powder
- 1 teaspoon oregano, dried
- ¼ teaspoon garlic powder
- 1 teaspoon rosemary, dried
- ½ teaspoon onion powder

How To:

1. Add pecans, oil, basil, chili powder, oregano, garlic powder, onion powder, rosemary and toss well.
2. Transfer to Slow Cooker and cook on LOW for 2 hours.
3. Divide between bowls and serve.
4. Enjoy!

Nutrition (Per Serving)

- Calories: 152
- Fat: 3g
- Carbohydrates: 11g
- Protein: 2g

Gentle Sweet Potato Tempura

Serving: 4
Prep Time: 15 minutes
Cook Time: 4 minutes
Ingredients:

- 2 whole eggs
- ½ teaspoon salt
- 3/4 cup ice water + 3 tablespoons ice water
- ¾ cup all-purpose flour + 1 tablespoons all-purpose flour
- 2 cups oil
- 1 sweet potato, scrubbed and sliced into 1/8 inch slices

For sauce

- ¼ cup rice wine
- ¼ cup coconut aminos

How To:

1. Take a large bowl and beat in eggs until frothy.
2. Stir in salt, ice water, and flour, mix well until the batter is lumpy.
3. Take a frying pan and place over high heat, add oil and heat to 350 degrees F.
4. Dry-sweet potato slices and dip 3 slices at a time in the batter, let excess batter drip.
5. Fry until golden brown on both sides, each side should take about 2 minutes.
6. Live them out and drain excess oil, keep repeating until all potatoes are done.
7. Take a small bowl and whisk in rice wine, soy sauce and use it as a dipping sauce.
8. Enjoy!

Nutrition (Per Serving)

- Calories: 315
- Fat: 13g
- Carbohydrates: 35g
- Protein: 8g

Japanese Cucumber Sunomono

Serving: 4
Prep Time: 15 minutes + 60 minutes chill time
Cook Time: Nil
Ingredients:

- 2 large sized cucumbers
- 1/3 cup of vinegar, rice
- 4 heaped teaspoons of sugar, white
- 1 heaped teaspoon of salt
- 1 ½ teaspoons freshly minced ginger root
- Seeds of sesame as needed

How To:

1. Cut cucumbers in half, lengthwise.
2. Scoop out any large seeds, slice crosswise into thin slices.
3. Take a small sized bowl and add ginger, salt, sugar and vinegar.
4. Mix thoroughly and add the cucumbers in the bowl.
5. Mix well to coat the cucumbers well .
6. Let it chill for about 1 hour.
7. Spread sesame and enjoy!

Nutrition (Per Serving)

- Calories: 27
- Fat: 0.2g
- Carbohydrates: 6g
- Protein: 0.6g

Radish and Hash Brown Dish

Serving: 4
Prep Time: 15 minutes + 60 minutes chill time
Cook Time: Nil
Ingredients:

- 1 pound radish, shredded
- ½ teaspoon onion powder
- 1/3 cup parmesan, grated
- ½ teaspoon garlic powder
- 4 whole eggs
- Pepper to taste

How To:

1. Mix in radishes, pepper, onion, garlic powder, eggs, parmesan in bowl and stir well.
2. Arrange neatly on lined baking sheet.
3. Pre-heat your oven to 375 degrees F.
4. Transfer to oven and bake for 10 minutes.
5. Cut Hash Browns and enjoy!

Nutrition (Per Serving)

- Calories: 60
- Fat: 5g
- Carbohydrates: 5g
- Protein: 7g

Kid Friendly Popsicles

Serving: 4
Prep Time: 2 hours
Cook Time: 15 minutes
Ingredients:

- 1 ½ cups raspberries
- 2 cups water

How To:

1. Take a pan and add water and raspberries.
2. Heat over medium heat.
3. Bring the water to a boil and reduce heat.
4. Simmer for 15 minutes.
5. Remove from the heat and pour mix into ice cube tray.
6. Add popsicle stick in each and chill for 2 hours.
7. Serve and enjoy!

Nutrition (Per Serving)

- Calories: 58
- Fat: 0.4g
- Carbohydrates: 0g
- Protein: 1.4g

Elegant Mango Compote

Serving: 4
Prep Time: 10 minutes
Cook Time: 10 minutes
Ingredients:

- 4 cups mango, peeled and cubed
- 1 cup orange juice
- 6 tablespoons palm sugar
- 3 tablespoons lime juice

How To:

1. Add mango, lime juice, orange juice, sugar to your Instant Pot.
2. Lock the lid and cook on LOW pressure for 10 minutes.
3. Release the pressure naturally over 10 minutes.
4. Remove the lid and divide amongst serving bowls.
5. Enjoy!

Nutrition (Per Serving)

- Calories: 180
- Fat: 2g
- Carbohydrates: 12g
- Protein: 2g

Everyone's Favorite Apple Pie

Serving: 4
Prep Time: 10 minutes
Cook Time: 10 minutes
Ingredients:

- 5 apples, cored, peeled and roughly chopped
- ½ cup water
- 1 tablespoon maple syrup
- ½ a teaspoon nutmeg, ground
- 2 teaspoon cinnamon powder
- 1 cup old-fashioned rolled oats
- 4 tablespoons fat-free butter, melted
- ¼ cup coconut sugar

How To:

1. Add apples to your Instant Pot alongside water, cinnamon, maple syrup and nutmeg.
2. Toss well.
3. Take a bowl and add butter, oats, sugar and whisk.
4. Spread over apple mix.
5. Lock the lid and cook on HIGH pressure for 10 minutes.
6. Release the pressure naturally over 10 minutes.
7. Open the lid and transfer to serving plates.
8. Serve and enjoy!

Nutrition (Per Serving)

- Calories: 200
- Fat: 6g
- Carbohydrates: 11g
- Protein: 7g

Plum and Apple Medley

Serving: 4
Prep Time: 10 minutes
Cook Time: 15 minutes
Ingredients:

- 1 plum, chopped, stone removed
- 1 apple, cored and cubed
- 2 tablespoons avocado oil
- 2 tablespoons coconut sugar
- 1 cup apple juice
- ½ teaspoon cinnamon powder
- ¼ cup coconut, shredded

How To:

1. Add plum, apple, sugar, oil, apple juice, cinnamon and coconut to your Instant Pot.
2. Toss well and lock the lid.
3. Cook on HIGH pressure for 15 minutes.
4. Release the pressure naturally over 10 minutes.
5. Divide amongst serving bowls and serve.
6. Enjoy!

Nutrition (Per Serving)

- Calories: 202
- Fat: 8g
- Carbohydrates: 12g
- Protein: 7g

Jalapeno Crisp For Keto Goers

Serving: 20
Prep Time: 10 minutes
Cook Time: 1 hour 15 minutes
Ingredients:

- 1 cup sesame seeds
- 1 cup sunflower seeds
- 1 cup flaxseeds
- ½ cup hulled hemp seeds
- 3 tablespoons Psyllium husk
- 1 teaspoon salt
- 1 teaspoon baking powder
- 2 cups water

How To:

1. Pre-heat your oven to 350 degrees F.
2. Take your blender and add seeds, baking powder, salt and Psyllium husk.
3. Blend well until a sand-like texture appears.
4. Stir in water and mix until a batter forms.
5. Allow the batter to rest for 10 minutes until a dough like thick mixture forms.
6. Pour the dough onto cookie sheet lined up with parchment paper.
7. Spread evenly, making sure that it has a ¼ inch thickness all around.
8. Bake for 75 minutes in the oven.
9. Remove and cut into 20 spices.
10. Allow them to cool for 30 minutes and enjoy!

Nutrition (Per Serving)

- Calories: 156
- Fat: 13g
- Carbohydrates: 2g
- Protein: 5g

Spicy Chicken Fingers

Prep Time: 20 minutes
Cooking Time: 30 minutes
Serving: 4
Ingredients:

- 1 ¼ pounds, skinless boneless chicken breast tenders
- ¼ teaspoon salt 1/8 teaspoon fresh ground black pepper
- 3 cups brown rice cereal
- ½ cup honey
- 2 teaspoons sriracha

How To:

1. Pre-heat your oven to 375 degrees F.
2. Take a baking sheet and coat with cooking spray.
3. Sprinkle both sides of chicken with salt and pepper.
4. Transfer brown rice cereal in a re-sealable bag and use rolling pin to crush cereal into pieces.
5. Pour crushed cereal into a large bowl.
6. Take a medium bowl and whisk in honey and sriracha.
7. Dip chicken tenders in honey mix, then dredge in cereal mix.
8. Place tenders on baking sheet, leaving about ½ inch gap between each tender.
9. Bake for 30 minutes until the internal temperature reaches 165 degrees F.
10. Serve and enjoy!

Nutrition (Per Serving)

- Calories: 331
- Fat: 4g
- Carbohydrates: 41g
- Protein: 33g

Lovely Carrot Cake

Prep Time: 3 hours 15 minutes
Cooking Time: Nil
Serving: 6
Ingredients:
For Cashew Frosting

- 2 tablespoons lemon juice
- 2 cups cashews, soaked
- 2 tablespoons coconut oil, melted
- 1/3 cup maple syrup
- water

For Cake

- 1 cup pineapple, dried and chopped
- 2 carrots, chopped
- 1 ½ cups coconut flour
- 1 cup dates, pitted
- ½ cup dry coconut
- ½ teaspoon cinnamon

How To:

1. Add cashews, lemon juice, maple syrup, coconut oil, apple and pulse well.
2. Transfer to a bowl and keep it on the side.
3. Add carrots to your processor and pulse a few times.
4. Add flour, dates, pineapple, coconut, cinnamon and pulse.
5. Pour half of the mixture into a spring form pan and spread well.
6. Add 1/3 of the cashew frosting and spread evenly.
7. Add remaining cake batter and spread the frosting.
8. Place in your freezer until it is hard.
9. Cut and serve.
10. Enjoy!

Nutrition (Per Serving)

- Calories: 140
- Fat: 4g
- Carbohydrates: 8g
- Protein: 4g

Grilled Peach with Honey Yogurt Dressing

Prep Time: 10 minutes
Cooking Time: 5 minutes
Serving: 6
Ingredients:

- 2 large peaches, ripe and halved
- 2 tablespoons honey
- 1/8 teaspoon cinnamon
- ¼ cut vanilla Greek yogurt, fat free

How To:

1. Prepare your outdoor grill and heat on low heat.
2. Grill your peaches on indirect heat until they are tender, it should take about 2-4 minutes each side.
3. Take a bowl and mix in yogurt and cinnamon.
4. Drizzle honey mix on top and enjoy!

Nutrition (Per Serving)

- Calories: 140
- Fat: 4g
- Carbohydrates: 8g
- Protein: 4g

Hearty Carrot Cookies

Prep Time: 10 minutes
Cooking Time: 15 minutes
Serving: 6
Ingredients:

- ½ cup packed light brown sugar
- ½ cup sugar
- ½ cup oil
- ½ cup apple sauce
- 2 whole eggs
- 1 cup flour
- 1 teaspoon vanilla
- 1 teaspoon baking soda
- 1 cup whole wheat flour
- ¼ teaspoon salt
- ½ teaspoon ground nutmeg
- 1 teaspoon cinnamon, ground
- 1 ½ cups carrots, grated
- 1 cup golden raisin
- 2 cups rolled oats, raw

How To:

1. Pre-heat your oven to about 350 degrees F.
2. Take a bowl and mix in applesauce, oil, sugar, vanilla and eggs.
3. Take another bowl and mix in the dry ingredients.
4. Blend the dry ingredients into the bowl with wet mixture.
5. Stir in carrots and raisins to the mix.
6. Take a greased cookie sheet and drop in the mixture spoon by spoon.
7. Transfer to oven and bake for 15 minutes until you have a golden brown texture.
8. Serve and enjoy!

Nutrition (Per Serving)

- Calories: 140
- Fat: 4g
- Carbohydrates: 8g
- Protein: 4g

Milky Pudding

Prep Time: 10 minutes
Cooking Time: 5-10 minutes + chill time
Serving: 6
Ingredients:

- 3 tablespoons cornstarch
- ½ teaspoon vanilla
- 1/3 cup chocolate chips
- 2 cups non-fat milk
- 1/8 teaspoon salt
- 2 tablespoons salt
- 2 tablespoons sugar

How To:

1. Take a medium sized bowl and add cocoa powder, cornstarch, salt, sugar and mix well.
2. Whisk in the milk.
3. Place over medium heat and keep heating until thick and bubbly.
4. Remove the mixture from heat and stir in vanilla and chocolate chips.
5. Keep mixing until the chips are melted and you have a smooth pudding.
6. Pour into a large sized dish and let it chill.
7. Serve and enjoy!

Nutrition:

- Calories: 140
- Fat: 4g
- Carbohydrates: 8g
- Protein: 4g

Fresh Honey Strawberries with Yogurt

Prep Time: 10 minutes
Cooking Time: 5-10 minutes + chill time
Serving: 6
Ingredients:

- 4 tablespoons almond, sliced and toasted
- 3 cups yogurt, low fat
- 4 teaspoons honey
- 1 pint fresh strawberries

How To:

1. Take your strawberries and wash under water, clean well.
2. Cut into quarters.
3. Take your serving dishes and add ¾ cup yogurt into each dish.
4. Divide strawberries among the dishes.
5. Top each dish with honey, sliced almonds.
6. Serve and enjoy!

Nutrition:

- Calories: 140
- Fat: 4g
- Carbohydrates: 8g
- Protein: 4g

Conclusion

I can't express how honored I am to think that you found my book interesting and informative enough to read it through to the end.

I thank you again for purchasing this book, and I hope that you had as much fun reading it as I had writing it.

I bid you farewell and encourage you to move forward with your Dash Diet journey!

Made in the USA
Middletown, DE
08 December 2019